Lean and Green Cookbook 2021

550-Day Tasty and Healthy Recipes to Help You Keep Healthy and Lose Weight.
With 4, 2 & 1 and 5 &1 Meal Plan

Leticia Hearn

Table of Contents

Introduction

Do you want to try something new, different and effective to achieve good health and active metabolism? Then here comes a fairly new concept known as the Lean and green diet. This dietary regime takes a whole new approach and suggests weight loss through multiple measures taken at a time. The diet is essentially restrictive, and it also promotes the use of food fueling to compensate for the reduced caloric intake and to meet all the nutritional needs. Well, in this cookbook, you will learn all about the basic concept of the fueling based diet, the lean and green diet approach, and its different weight loss programs. There are various factors that work together to make the lean and green diet plan effective for weight loss; all such factors are thoroughly discussed in the first part of the book.

The content of this cookbook comes from my own experience of trying the lean and green diet and finding it quite effective for weight loss. I had never tried a meal replacement diet before, so for me, it was a first-hand experience of trying this weight loss program. Initially, I tried the 3x3 lean and green diet plan, and the results came out to be pretty satisfying. From that point, I tried its other plans as well. With Lean and green diet I not only managed to lose some weight, but it brought me good health as well. Let's see how you can put this dietary approach up to its best use. The part of this book is designed you introduce the basics of the lean and green diet, where you will get to know about the lean and green meals and food that are suitable to prepare its weight loss meal plan. The second part of this book will provide you with several recipes to introduce and incorporate all the lean and green ingredients into your diet while adding a variety of flavours and aromas.

Lean and Green diet

Lean and green diet is basically a weight loss or weight maintenance program that suggests the use of a lean and green meal along with processed food called "fueling." The diet says to add these nutritional Fuelings to the diet while controlling the overall caloric intake. The fueling is actually powdered food, which is mixed with liquid like water and then added to the diet as a part of routine meals. Besides consuming these fueling, the dieters are also suggested to exercise 30 minutes daily to lose weight. By trying fueling as a substitute for real food, you can curb the carb and sugar intake and can manage your caloric intake as well. How much Fuelings to consume, how much food to eat, and what to eat on this dietary regime depends on the type of weight loss plan you are going for. However, on this diet, the overall calorie intake for adults is reduced to 800 to 1000 per day, which lets you lose about 12 lbs of weight per 12 weeks on average.

What do you eat on the lean and green diet?

The following are the food items that you can opt for on this diet plan:

1. **Meat:**

The lean and green diet only allows 85 per cent of lean meat on a diet; whether it is chicken, beef, turkey, lamb, pork, and ground meat, it all has to be lean. Lean meat has lower fat content, which makes it great to keep the caloric intake in control.

2. **Seafood:**

Seafood is best to have on any weight loss regime because it is free from saturated fats and brings a lot of nutritional value to the table. You can have all types of fishes and seafood on this diet, including halibut, salmon, trout, lobster, tuna, shrimp, crab, and scallops, etc.

3. **Eggs:**

Eggs are rich in protein, and they are low in carbs; that's what makes eggs the right for this diet.

4. **Soy products:**

In soy products, tofu is the only product that is allowed on the lean and green diet because it is processed, and the caloric content is suitable for the lean diet.

5. **Fats:**

Not all fats are healthy, and there are a handful of options that you must try on this diet that includes most of the vegetable olive oil, walnut oil, canola oil, flaxseed oil. Other fats sources that can be incorporated into this diet include nuts and seeds, reduced-fat margarine, and olives.

6. Low carb vegetables:

All low-carb vegetables are a suitable fit for the Lean and green diet. So, except potatoes, yams, sweet potatoes, yellow squash, and beetroots, you can try every other vegetable on this diet, including spinach, cabbage, collard greens, cucumbers, mushrooms, celery, onion, tomatoes, garlic, ginger, eggplant, cauliflower, broccoli, bell peppers, zucchini, and spaghetti squash, etc.

7. Sugar-free snacks:

Snacks are usually loaded with carbs and sugar, so they must be avoided most of the time. But you have snacks in some amounts, then only try the sugar-free and low-carb snacks.

8. Sugar-free beverages:

In beverages, there are limited options as well. For the most part of this diet, water is the most recommended drink since it is zero caloric and comes with several health advantages. Besides that, you can have unsweetened almond milk, coconut milk, sugar-free tea, coffee

9. Condiments and seasonings:

In condiments and seasonings, there are no such restrictions; from dried herbs to salt, lemon juice, ground and whole spices, lime juice, yellow mustard, soy sauce, and salsa, you can use any. Whereas in syrups and sauces, stay from the sugar-rich varieties and try the sugar-free syrups, low-carb sweeteners, sugar-free ketchup and barbecue sauce, etc.

Foods to avoid

- All fried foods are off the list for the lean and green diet, whether it is the fried fish, meat, poultry, fruits, vegetables, or fried desserts.
- The high carb refined grain items are also not a suitable option for this diet; such products include pasta, white bread, flour tortillas, biscuits, pancakes crackers, white rice, cakes, cookies, pastries, and other similar baked goods.
- Saturated fats from butter or solid shortening are also not the right fit for this diet.
- Milk, yogurt, and cheese are termed whole-fat dairy items, and they must also be avoided.
- All varieties of alcohol are strictly forbidden on this diet.
- All sweetened beverages like soda drinks, sports drinks, fruit juices, energy drinks, flavored milk, and sweetened tea, etc., are also not allowed for this diet.

Breakfast Recipes

Cauliflower Breakfast Casserole

Prep Time: 10 minutes.
Cook Time: 55 minutes.
Serves: 8

Ingredients:

- 8 ounces turkey sausage, cooked
- ¼ cup onion, chopped
- 2 cups cauliflower florets
- ½ teaspoon Jalapeno Seasoning
- ¼ teaspoon salt
- ¼ teaspoon black pepper
- 6 turkey bacon slices, cooked and chopped
- 2 cups Mexican cheese, shredded
- 8 large eggs
- 16 ounces egg whites
- ¼ cup almond milk

Preparation:

1. At 350 degrees F, preheat your oven.
2. Grease a baking dish with cooking spray.
3. Saute turkey sausage in a skillet until golden brown.
4. Saute onions and cauliflower in a same skillet until golden.
5. Stir in black pepper, salt, jalapeno seasoning then mix well.
6. Sread the cauliflower mixture in the prepared baking dish.
7. Top this mixture with cheese and bacon.
8. Beat egg whites with eggs and almond milk in a bowl.
9. Pour this mixture over the turkey mixture.
10. Bake for 45 minutes in the oven.
11. Garnish with green onions.
12. Serve warm.

Serving Suggestion: Enjoy this breakfast casserole with a refreshing smoothie.

Variation Tip: Add some chopped or shredded zucchini to the casserole.

Nutritional Information Per Serving:
Calories 244 | Fat 7.9g |Sodium 704mg | Carbs 19g | Fiber 2g | Sugar 14g | Protein 14g

Quinoa Pudding

Prep Time: 10 minutes.
Cook Time: 25 minutes.
Serves: 4

Ingredients:

- 1 cup quinoa
- 4 cups coconut milk
- 1/3 cup maple syrup
- 1 ½ teaspoons vanilla extract
- 1 teaspoon cinnamon
- 1/4 teaspoon salt

Preparation:

1. Mix quinoa, milk, maple, vanilla, cinnamon and salt in a saucepan.
2. Boil this mixture, reduce the heat and cook for 25 minutes.
3. Garnish with your favorite toppings.
4. Serve warm.

Serving Suggestion: Serve this pudding with toasted bread slices.

Variation Tip: Add chopped berries and nuts to the pudding.

Nutritional Information Per Serving:
Calories 214 | Fat 5.1g |Sodium 231mg | Carbs 31g | Fiber 5g | Sugar 2.1g | Protein 7g

Cranberry Sweet Potato Muffins

Prep Time: 15 minutes.
Cook Time: 20 minutes.
Serves: 4

Ingredients:

- 2 tablespoons butter, melted
- 1/4 cup brown sugar
- 1 egg
- 1 teaspoon vanilla
- 1/4 cup skim milk
- 1/2 cup curd cottage cheese
- 1/2 cup cooked sweet potato, mashed
- 3/4 cup white whole wheat flour
- 1 teaspoon baking powder
- 1 cup fresh cranberries

Preparation:

1. Mix all the ingredients for batter in a bowl until smooth.
2. Stir in cranberries then divide the batter into muffin cups.
3. Bake for 20 minutes at 350 degrees F.
4. Allow the cranberries to cool then serve.

Serving Suggestion: Enjoy these muffins with a refreshing smoothie.

Variation Tip: Add some riasins to the muffins.

Nutritional Information Per Serving:
Calories 225 | Fat 9g |Sodium 118mg | Carbs 35.4g | Fiber 2.9g | Sugar 15g | Protein 6.5g

Quinoa Bars

Prep Time: 15 minutes.
Cook Time: 20 minutes.
Serves: 6

Ingredients:

- 1 cup whole wheat flour
- 1 ½ cup cooked quinoa
- 2 cup oats
- 1/2 cup nuts, chopped
- 1 teaspoon cinnamon
- 1 teaspoon baking soda
- 2 tablespoons chia seeds
- 2/3 cup peanut butter
- 1/2 cup honey
- 2 eggs
- 2/3 cup applesauce
- 1teaspoons vanilla
- 1/2 teaspoon salt
- 1/3 cup craisins
- 1/3 cup chocolate chips

Preparation:

1. Mix quinoa with honey, peanut butter, eggs, vanilla, applesauce in a small bowl.
2. Stir in rest of the ingredients then mix well.
3. Spread this mixture in a 9x13 greased baking dish.
4. Bake for 20 minutes at 375 degrees F then cut into bars.
5. Serve.

Serving Suggestion: Enjoy these bars with a strawberry smoothie.

Variation Tip: Add some goji berries to the bars.

Nutritional Information Per Serving:

Calories 163 | Fat 2.5g |Sodium 15.6mg | Carbs 49.5g | Fiber 7.6g | Sugar 28g | Protein 3.5g

Buckwheat Crepes

Prep Time: 15 minutes.
Cook Time: 10 minutes.
Serves: 4

Ingredients:

- 2/3 cup buckwheat flour
- 1/3 cup whole wheat flour
- 2 eggs
- 1 ¼ cup skim milk
- 1 tablespoon honey
- Fruit and Greek yogurt, for filling

Preparation:

1. Mix flours with eggs, milk, and honey in a bowl until smooth.
2. Set a nonstick skillet over medium heat.
3. Add a ¼ cup batter into the skillet, spread it evenly then cook for 2 minutes per side.

4. Transfer the crepe to a plate and then cook the remaining batter in the same way.
5. Garnish with fruits and yogurt.
6. Serve.

Serving Suggestion: Enjoy these crepes with a blueberry smoothie.

Variation Tip: Add some blueberries to the crepes filling.

Nutritional Information Per Serving:
Calories 112 | Fat 25g |Sodium 132mg | Carbs 44g | Fiber 3.9g | Sugar 3g | Protein 8.9g

Oatmeal Pancakes

Prep Time: 10 minutes.
Cook Time: 10 minutes.
Serves: 6

Ingredients:

- 2/3 cup Greek Yogurt
- 3 tablespoons skim milk
- 1 tablespoon applesauce
- 1 egg
- 1/2 cup white whole wheat flour
- 3/4 cup oats, crushed
- 1 teaspoon baking powder
- 1/2 teaspoon baking soda
- 1 tablespoon ground flaxseed
- 1 teaspoon cinnamon

Preparation:

1. Mix flours and rest of the ingredients in a bowl until smooth.
2. Set a hot griddle over medium heat.
3. Pour a ladle of battter over the griddle and cook the pancake for 2 mintues per side.
4. Transfer to a plate and cook remaining pancakes in the same manner.
5. Serve warm.

Serving Suggestion: Enjoy these pancakes with a spinach smoothie.

Variation Tip: Add chopped nuts to the batter.

Nutritional Information Per Serving:
Calories 190 | Fat 15g |Sodium 595mg | Carbs 11g | Fiber 3g | Sugar 12g | Protein 9g

Blueberry Muffins

Prep Time: 15 minutes.
Cook Time: 30 minutes.
Serves: 4

Ingredients:

- 2 tablespoons butter, melted
- 1 cup fresh blueberries
- 1/4 cup sugar
- 1 egg
- 1 teaspoon vanilla
- 1/4 cup skim milk
- 1/2 cup curd cottage cheese
- 1/2 cup cooked sweet potato, mashed
- 3/4 cup whole wheat flour
- 1 teaspoon baking powder

Preparation:

1.   Mix sweet potato mash with all the ingredients except cranberries in a bowl until smooth.
2.   Fold in blueberries then mix evenly.
3.   Divide the batter into the muffin tray and bake for 30 minutes at 350 degrees F.
4.   Serve.

Serving Suggestion: Enjoy these muffins with a strawberry smoothie.

Variation Tip: Add raisins to the muffin batter.

Nutritional Information Per Serving:

Calories 197 | Fat 15g |Sodium 202mg | Carbs 58.5g | Fiber 4g | Sugar 1g | Protein 7.3g

Berry Quinoa

Prep Time: 10 minutes.
Cook Time: 20 minutes.
Serves: 4

Ingredients:

- ¼ cup quinoa, rinsed
- 1/2 cup almond milk
- 1/2 cup berries
- 1 dash cinnamon
- 1/2 teaspoon vanilla

Toppings

- Nuts
- Fruit
- Chocolate chips
- Nut butter
- Agave/honey

Preparation:

1. Mix quinoa with milk, vanilla, cinnamon and berries in a saucepan.
2. Cook to a boil, reduce its heat and cook for 20 minutes until liquid is absorbed.
3. Garnish with desired toppings.
4. Serve.

Serving Suggestion: Enjoy this quinoa with a cranberry muffin.

Variation Tip: Add roasted nuts to the quinoa.

Nutritional Information Per Serving:
Calories 163 | Fat 6.5g |Sodium 548mg | Carbs 3.4g | Fiber 2g | Sugar 1g | Protein 2g

Snacks and Appetizer Recipes

Celery Salad

Prep Time: 5 minutes.
Cook Time: 0 minutes.
Serves: 2

Ingredients:

- 1 cup celery, chopped
- 1 tablespoon mint, chopped
- 1 teaspoon lemon juice
- 1 teaspoon olive oil

Preparation:

1. Mix celery with mint, lemon juice and olive oil in a salad bowl.
2. Serve.

Serving Suggestion: Serve this salad with grilled shrimp.

Variation Tip: Drizzle dried herbs and cumin on top.

Nutritional Information Per Serving:
Calories 148 | Fat 22g |Sodium 350mg | Carbs 32.2g | Fiber 0.7g | Sugar 1g | Protein 4.3g

Taco Salad

Prep Time: 5 minutes.

Cook Time: 0 minutes.

Serves: 2

Ingredients:

- 5 ounces ground turkey
- 1 tablespoon taco seasoning
- 2 tablespoons salsa
- 1 cup romaine lettuce
- 1 cup iceberg lettuce
- 1/2 cup diced tomatoes
- 1 tablespoon water

Preparation:

1. Saute turkey with taco seasoning in a skillet until golden brown.
2. Transfer to a salad bowl and stir in salsa, lettuces, tomatoes and water.
3. Mix well and serve.

Serving Suggestion: Serve this salad with grilled chicken.

Variation Tip: Drizzle black pepper ground on top before serving.

Nutritional Information Per Serving:

Calories 345 | Fat 9g |Sodium 48mg | Carbs 14g | Fiber 1g | Sugar 2g | Protein 20g

Yogurt Trail Mix Bars

Prep Time: 15 minutes.

Cook Time: 0 minutes.

Serves: 4

Ingredients:

- 2 cups Greek yogurt
- 1 ½ cups fruit
- 1/2 cup almonds, chopped
- 3/4 cup granola
- 1/4 cup chocolate chips

Preparation:

1. Mix yogurt with fruit, almonds, granola and chocolate chips in a bowl.
2. Spread this mixture in a shallow tray and freeze for 1 hour.
3. Cut the mixture into bars.
4. Serve.

Serving Suggestion: Serve these bars with a berry compote.

Variation Tip: Pour melted chococlate on top and then slice to serve.

Nutritional Information Per Serving:

Calories 204 | Fat 3g |Sodium 216mg | Carbs 17g | Fiber 3g | Sugar 4g | Protein 11g

Curried Tuna Salad

Prep Time: 15 minutes.
Cook Time: 0 minutes.
Serves: 2

Ingredients:

- 2 cans of tuna, drained
- ¼ cup hummus
- ¼ cup avocado, smashed
- ½ cup apple, chopped
- ¼ cup onion, diced
- 1 tablespoon lemon juice
- 2 teaspoons curry powder
- 1/2 teaspoon dry mustard powder

Preparation:

1. Mix tuna with rest of the ingredients in a salad bowl.
2. Serve fresh.

Serving Suggestion: Serve this salad with grilled shrimp.

Variation Tip: Drizzle shredded coconut on top before serving.

Nutritional Information Per Serving:

Calories 280 | Fat 9g |Sodium 318mg | Carbs 19g | Fiber 5g | Sugar 3g | Protein 17g

Tuna Quinoa Cakes

Prep Time: 15 minutes.
Cook Time: 20 minutes.
Serves: 4

Ingredients:

- 1/2 cup cooked sweet potato, mashed
- 2 cans tuna, drained
- 3/4 cup cooked quinoa
- 1/4 cup green onion, chopped
- 2 garlic cloves, minced
- 1 tablespoon lemon juice
- 1 egg
- 1/4 cup plain yogurt
- 1 tablespoon mustard
- 1/2 teaspoon cayenne pepper
- 1 teaspoon paprika
- 1/2 cup breadcrumbs

Preparation:

1. In a small bowl, combine the tuna and sweet potato and mix well.
2. Add remaining ingredients and stir until well combined.
3. Make 6 patties out of this mixture.
4. Place the patties in a greased baking sheet and bake for 20 minutes at 400 degrees F.
5. Flip the patties once cooked half way through.
6. Serve warm.

Serving Suggestion: Serve the cakes with cream cheese dip on the side.

Variation Tip: Add shredded parmesan before cooking.

Nutritional Information Per Serving:

Calories 273 | Fat 8g |Sodium 146mg | Carbs 18g | Fiber 5g | Sugar 1g | Protein 7g

Taco Cups

Prep Time: 15 minutes.
Cook Time: 25 minutes.
Serves: 4

Ingredients:

- 2 Sargento cheese slices
- 4 ounces lean ground beef
- 1 teaspoon taco seasoning

Toppings:

- Lettuce and tomatoes
- 1 tablespoon sour cream

Preparation:

1. At 375 degrees F, preheat your oven.
2. Saute beef in a skillet for 5 minutes.
3. Stir in taco seasoning then mix well.
4. Layer a baking sheet with wax papper.
5. Place cheese slices in the baking sheet and bake for 7 minutes in the oven.
6. Allow the cheese to cool and then place each cheese round in the muffin tray.
7. Press the cheese into cups and divide the beef into these cups.
8. Garnish with desired toppings.
9. Serve warm.

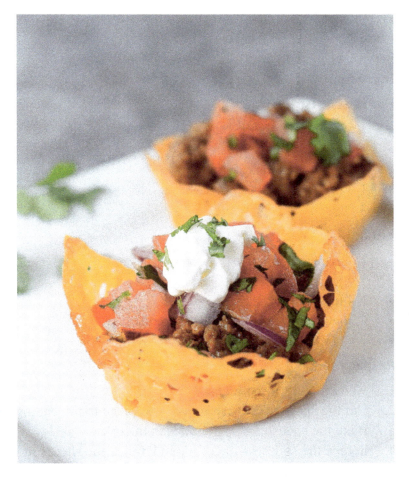

Serving Suggestion: Serve the cups with guacamole.

Variation Tip: Add shredded cheese to the filling.

Nutritional Information Per Serving:
Calories 240 | Fat 25g |Sodium 244mg | Carbs 16g | Fiber 1g | Sugar 1g | Protein 27g

Caprese Spaghetti Squash Nests

Prep Time: 15 minutes.

Cook Time: 1 hr 35 minutes.

Serves: 4

Ingredients:

For the Nests:

- 1 medium spaghetti squash
- 1/4 teaspoon salt
- 1/4 teaspoon black pepper
- 1/4 teaspoon garlic powder
- 3 tablespoons egg whites

Filling:

- 1 cup cherry tomatoes
- 1/4 teaspoon salt
- 1/4 teaspoon black pepper
- 4 ounces mozzarella cheese, shredded
- 1/4 cup basil, chopped

Preparation:

1. At 375 degrees F, preheat your oven.
2. Cut the spaghetti squash in half and place in the baking sheet.
3. Bake the squash for 45 minutes in the oven.
4. Scrape the squash with a fork and divide the shreds in the muffin tray.
5. Beat egg whites with garlic powder, black pepper and salt.
6. Divide this liquid mixture into the muffin cups, make a nest at the center of each and bake for 20 minutes.
7. Spread tomatoes in a baking sheet and bake for 20 minutes in the oven.
8. Divide the roasted tomaotes in the spaghetti squash and top them with cheese and rest of the ingredients.
9. Bake for 10 minutes in the oven.
10. Serve warm.

Serving Suggestion: Serve the nests with spinach or cream cheese dip.

Variation Tip: Add shredded parmesan on top.

Nutritional Information Per Serving:

Calories 282 | Fat 4g |Sodium 232mg | Carbs 7g | Fiber 1g | Sugar 0g | Protein 14g

Fire Cracker Shrimp

Prep Time: 15 minutes.
Cook Time: 6 minutes.
Serves: 4

Ingredients:

- 11 ounces raw shrimp, peeled
- 2 tablespoons Apricot Preserves
- 1 teaspoon lite soy sauce
- ½ teaspoon sriracha sauce
- 1 teaspoon sesame oil

Preparation:

1. Place apricot in a small bowl and heat for 20 seconds in the microwave.
2. Mix oil, sriracha sauce, soy sauce and apricot mixture in a bowl.
3. Thread the shrimp on the wooden skewers and brush them with apricot mixture.
4. Grill these skewers for 3 minutes per side.
5. Serve warm.

Serving Suggestion: Serve the shrimp with zucchini fries.

Variation Tip: Add crumbled cheese on top.

Nutritional Information Per Serving:
Calories 229 | Fat 5g |Sodium 510mg | Carbs 37g | Fiber 5g | Sugar 4g | Protein 21g

Crispy Zucchini Chips

Prep Time: 15 minutes.

Cook Time: 4 hrs.

Serves: 4

Ingredients:

- 1 ½ cups zucchini
- 1 teaspoon olive oil
- 1/8 teaspoons salt

Preparation:

1. At 200 degrees F, preheat your oven.
2. Layer a baking sheet with wax paper and grease with cooking spray.
3. Spread the zucchini slices in the baking sheet and bake for 4 hours.
4. Flip the zucchinin once cooked half way through.
5. Serve warm.

Serving Suggestion: Serve the chips with tomato sauce.

Variation Tip: Drizzle black pepper on top before serving.

Nutritional Information Per Serving:

Calories 101 | Fat 7g |Sodium 269mg | Carbs 5g | Fiber 4g | Sugar 12g | Protein 1g

Baked Kale Chips

Prep Time: 15 minutes.
Cook Time: 15 minutes.
Serves: 4

Ingredients:

- 4 ½ cups kale
- 1 tablespoon olive oil
- 1/4 teaspoon salt

Preparation:

1.   At 450 degree F, preheat your oven.
2.   Layer a baking sheet with parchment paper.
3.   Toss the kale leaves with salt, and olive oil in the baking sheet.
4.   Spread them evenly then bake for 15 minutes in the oven.
5.   Serve.

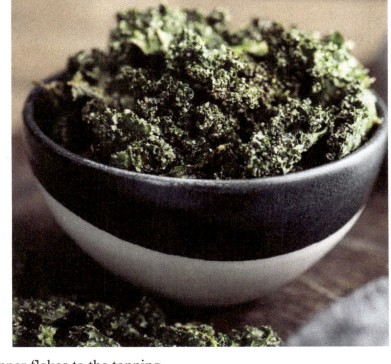

Serving Suggestion: Serve these chips with chilli garlic sauce.

Variation Tip: Add some paprika or red pepper flakes to the topping.

Nutritional Information Per Serving:

Calories 118 | Fat 11g |Sodium 110mg | Carbs 4g | Fiber 5g | Sugar 3g | Protein 1g

Grilled Buffalo Shrimp

Prep Time: 15 minutes.

Cook Time: 8 minutes.

Serves: 4

Ingredients:

- 11 ounce raw shrimp, peeled
- 1/4 cup Frank's Hot Sauce
- 1 tablespoon butter

Preparation:

1. Mix butter with hot sauce in a bowl.
2. Thread the shrimp on the skewers and brush them with butter mixture.
3. Grill these skewers for 2 minutes per side while basting with butter sauce.
4. Serve warm.

Serving Suggestion: Serve the shrimps with tomato ketchup.

Variation Tip: Coat the shrimp in breadcrumbs before cooking.

Nutritional Information Per Serving:

Calories 275 | Fat 16g | Sodium 255mg | Carbs 1g | Fiber 1.2g | Sugar 5g | Protein 19g

Poultry Mains

Sheet Pan Chicken

Prep Time: 15 minutes.

Cook Time: 18 minutes.

Serves: 4

Ingredients:

- 1 ¾ pounds boneless chicken breasts, diced
- Salt, to taste
- 1 pound broccoli crowns
- 1 medium red bell pepper
- 2 tablespoons olive oil
- ¼ cup peanut butter
- 1 tablespoon tamari
- 1 tablespoon rice vinegar
- 1 tablespoon honey
- juice from ½ lime
- 3 tablespoons water
- 1 pinch of salt
- Sesame seeds
- Sliced green onions

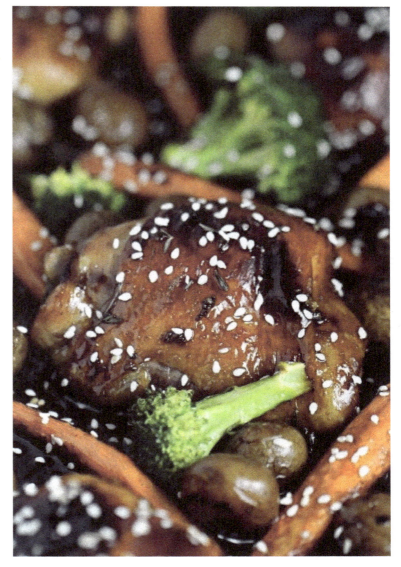

Preparation:

1. At 425 degrees F, preheat your oven.
2. Layer 2 baking sheets with wax paper and grease with cooking spray.
3. Toss chicken, veggies and all the ingredients in a large bowl.
4. Divide this mixture in the prepared baking seet.
5. Bake the mixture for 18 minutes in the oven.
6. Garnis whti sesame seeds and green onions.
7. Serve warm.

Serving Suggestion: Serve the chicken with a kale salad on the side.

Variation Tip: Coat the chicken with coconut shreds for a crispy texture.

Nutritional Information Per Serving:

Calories 384 | Fat 15g |Sodium 587mg | Carbs 8g | Fiber 1g | Sugar 5g | Protein 20g

Green Chicken Casserole

Prep Time: 15 minutes.
Cook Time: 25 minutes.
Serves: 6

Ingredients:

- 6 whole wheat tortillas
- 1 (15-oz) can white beans
- 1 (12-oz) bag cheese mexican blend, shredded
- 1 cup monterey jack cheese, shredded
- 1 (24-oz) jar salsa verde
- 2 (4-oz) cans of green hatch chiles
- 1 cup shredded salsa chicken
- 1 tablespoon dried oregano

TOPPINGS

- Greek Yogurt
- Guacamole
- Hot sauce
- Fresh cilantro

Preparation:

1. At 375 degrees F, preheat your oven.
2. Spread four tortilla halves in a 9x13 inches baking dish.
3. Top the tortillas with salsa verde to cover.
4. Mix beans with chile mixture and chicken in a bowl.
5. Sprread half of this mixture over the salsa verde.
6. Repeat the layers and top with cheese.
7. Bake for 25 mminutes in the oven at 375 degrees F.
8. Serve warm.

Serving Suggestion: Serve the casserole with roasted green beans.

Variation Tip: Add some sliced onion and spring onion to the casserole.

Nutritional Information Per Serving:
Calories 335 | Fat 5g |Sodium 422mg | Carbs 16g | Fiber 0g | Sugar 1g | Protein 25g

Broccoli Chicken Casserole

Prep Time: 15 minutes.

Cook Time: 20 minutes.

Serves: 4

Ingredients:

- 2 pounds boneless chicken breasts
- 1 tablespoon olive oil
- 2 10-ounce bags frozen cauliflower rice
- 1 (16-ounce) bag frozen broccoli cuts
- 2 large eggs, whisked
- 3 cups mozzarella cheese, shredded
- 2 teaspoons salt
- 2 teaspoons garlic powder
- 2 teaspoons onion powder
- 2 tablespoons butter, melted
- 1 cup Italian blend cheese, shredded

Preparation:

1. At 400 degrees F, preheat your oven.
2. Grease a baking dish with cooking spray.
3. Rub the chicken with oil, black pepper and salt then place in the baking sheet.
4. Bake the chicken breasts for 20 minutes.
5. Cook the cauliflower rice and broccoli as per the package's instructions.
6. Cut the baked chicken into cubes.
7. Mix chicken with rest of the ingredients in a bowl.
8. Spread this mixture in the baking dish and bake for 50 minutes in the oven.
9. Serve warm.

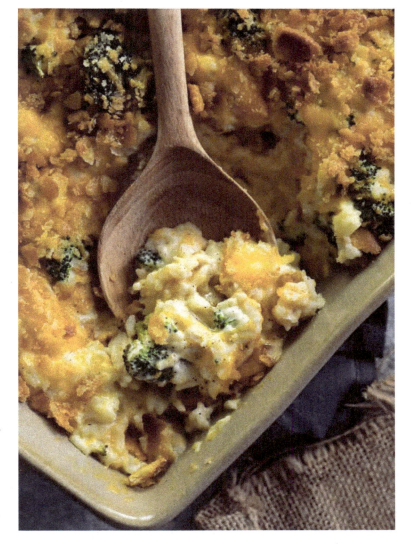

Serving Suggestion: Serve the casserole with roasted veggies.

Variation Tip: Add chopped carrots to the casserole.

Nutritional Information Per Serving:

Calories 369 | Fat 14g |Sodium 442mg | Carbs 13.3g | Fiber 0.4g | Sugar 2g | Protein 32.3g

Chicken with Green Beans

Prep Time: 15 minutes.

Cook Time: 11 minutes.

Serves: 4

Ingredients:

- 1 pound chicken breast cutlets
- 1 teaspoon salt, divided
- ½ teaspoon black pepper
- 2 tablespoons olive oil
- 6 cups green beans, trimmed
- 4 garlic cloves, sliced
- 1 teaspoon lemon zest, grated
- 1 teaspoon fresh thyme, chopped
- ¼ cup chicken broth
- ¼ cup dry white wine
- 1 tablespoon lemon juice
- ¼ cup pine nuts, toasted
- Lemon wedges for garnish

Preparation:

1. Season the chicken with black pepper, oil and salt.
2. Sear the chicken cutlets for 4 minutes per side in a skillet.
3. Sautte green beans with salt, oil and black pepper in a pan for 2 minutes.
4. Stir in wine, broth a nd lemon juie.
5. Cook for 1 minute then add chicken.
6. Garnish with pine nuts, lemon wedges and thyme.
7. Serve warm.

Serving Suggestion: Serve the chicken with fresh cucumber and couscous salad.

Variation Tip: Add some green peas to the mixture.

Nutritional Information Per Serving:

Calories 453 | Fat 2.4g |Sodium 216mg | Carbs 18g | Fiber 2.3g | Sugar 1.2g | Protein 23.2g

Cheddar Turkey Burgers

Prep Time: 15 minutes.

Cook Time: 14 minutes.

Serves: 4

Ingredients:

- 1 lb lean ground turkey
- 1 (1 ounce) envelope dry ranch dressing
- 1 cup cheddar cheese, shredded
- 1/4 cup green onion, chopped

Preparation:

1. Mix turkey ground with ranch dressing, cheese and green onion in a bowl.
2. Make six patties out of this mixture.
3. Sear each patties in a skillet for 7 minutes per side.
4. Serve warm.

Serving Suggestion: Serve the burgers with fresh herbs on top.

Variation Tip: Add some chopped bell pepper to the patties.

Nutritional Information Per Serving:

Calories 332 | Fat 18g |Sodium 611mg | Carbs 13.3g | Fiber 0g | Sugar g4 | Protein 38g

Turkey Taco Soup

Prep Time: 15 minutes.
Cook Time: 45 minutes.
Serves: 6

Ingredients:

- 1 ½ lbs. lean ground turkey
- 1 onion, diced
- 1 (1 ¼ ounces) package taco seasoning
- 1 (1 ounce) package ranch dressing seasoning
- 1 (14oz) can chicken broth
- 1 (4 ounces) can diced green chiles
- 1 (15 ½ ounces) can whole kernel corn
- 1 (15 ½ ounces)can pinto beans
- 1 (15 ounces) can refried beans
- 1 (14 ½ ounces) can diced tomatoes with green chiles
- 1 (14 ½ ounces) can mexican diced tomatoes

Preparation:

1. Saute onion and turkey in a skillet until golden brown.
2. Stir in rest of the ingredients and cook for 45 minutes.
3. Serve warm.

Serving Suggestion: Serve the soup with toasted bread slices.

Variation Tip: Add zucchini noodles to the soup.

Nutritional Information Per Serving:
Calories 354 | Fat 25g |Sodium 412mg | Carbs 22.3g | Fiber 0.2g | Sugar 1g | Protein 28.3g

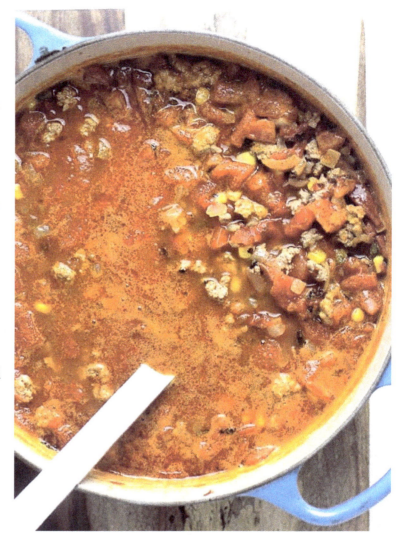

Chicken Zucchini

Prep Time: 15 minutes.
Cook Time: 30 minutes.

Serves: 4

Ingredients:

- 4 pieces of chicken breast
- 1 cup Zucchini, chopped
- 2 tablespoons shredded cheese
- 1 raw onion, chopped
- Salt, to taste
- Black pepper, to taste
- Oregano, to taste

Preparation:

1. At 450 degrees F, preheat your oven.
2. Place the chicken breast in a baking pan and drizzle oregano, black pepper and salt on top.
3. Drizzle cheese on top and cover the chicken with zucchini slices.
4. Bake this chicken for 30 minutes in the oven.
5. Serve warm.

Serving Suggestion: Serve the chicken with white rice or sweet potato salad.

Variation Tip: Add some zucchini noodles to the chicken.

Nutritional Information Per Serving:

Calories 405 | Fat 15g |Sodium 852mg | Carbs 7g | Fiber 2g | Sugar 2g | Protein 15g

Turkey Shepherds Pie

Prep Time: 15 minutes.
Cook Time: 30 minutes.
Serves: 4

Ingredients:

- 12 ounces lean ground turkey
- 2 cups cooked potatoes, mashed
- 1 cup frozen corn
- 1/2 cup tomatoes, diced
- 1/2 cup carrots, diced
- 1/2 cup zucchini, diced
- 1/4 cup onions, chopped
- 3 teaspoons garlic, minced
- salt and black pepper, to taste

Preparation:

1. Saute turkey with black pepper, salt, garlic, carrots, and onion in a skillet until golden brown.
2. Spread the turkey in a 9x12 inch baking pan.
3. Top it with tomatoes, zucchini, carrots, garlic and onion.
4. Add frozen corn and mashed potatoes on top.
5. Bake this casserole for 20 minutes in the oven at 350 degrees F.
6. Serve warm.

Serving Suggestion: Serve the pie with avocado tomato salad.

Variation Tip: Add boiled peas to the pie.

Nutritional Information Per Serving:
Calories 352 | Fat 14g |Sodium 220mg | Carbs 16g | Fiber 0.2g | Sugar 1g | Protein 26g

Turkey Broccoli

Prep Time: 15 minutes.
Cook Time: 20 minutes.
Serves: 4

Ingredients:

- 1 tablesepoon Dijon mustard
- 1 tablespoon whole grain mustard
- 1 cup chicken broth
- 4 teaspoons roasted garlic oil
- 4 cups broccoli florets
- 1 tablespoon garlic gusto seasoning
- 1½ lb boneless turkey breasts, diced
- 1 pinch dash of desperation seasoning

Preparation:

1. Mix broth with mustard in a bowl.
2. Saute broccoli with oil and garlic gusto in a skillet for 2 minutes.
3. Transfer the broccoli to a bowl.
4. Sear the turkey bites in the same pan for 5 minutes per side.
5. Reduce heat, and stir in mustard mixture and broccoli.
6. Cover and cook for 7 minutes on a simmer.
7. Serve warm.

Serving Suggestion: Serve the chicken with a spinach salad.

Variation Tip: Add chopped green beans to the mixture.

Nutritional Information Per Serving:
Calories 388 | Fat 8g |Sodium 339mg | Carbs 8g | Fiber 1g | Sugar 2g | Protein 33g

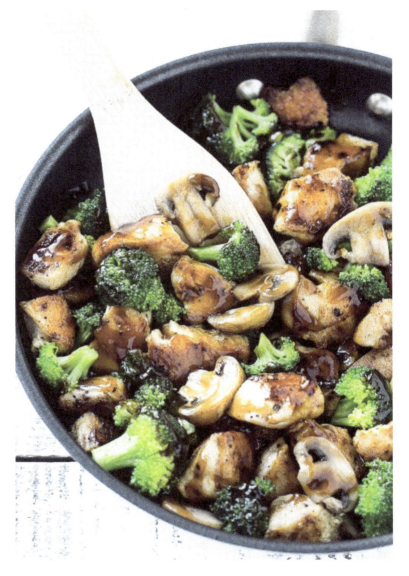

Baked Chicken Stuffed

Prep Time: 15 minutes.
Cook Time: 22 minutes.
Serves: 4

Ingredients:

- 4 chicken breast halves
- 4 ounces baby bella mushrooms
- 1/4 cup onion, chopped
- 1/2 teaspoon ground thyme
- 1/2 teaspoon salt
- 1/4 cup mozzarella cheese, shredded

Preparation:

1. At 350 degrees F, preheat your oven.
2. Layer a 9x13 inches baking dish with cooking oil.
3. Saute mushrooms, onions, salt and thyme in a skillet for 7 minutes.
4. Make a pocket in each chiekn breast and stuff each with the msurhoos mixture and cheese.
5. Place these chicken pockets in the baking dish.
6. Bake for 15 minutes in the oven.
7. Serve warm.

Serving Suggestion: Serve the chicken with steaming white rice.

Variation Tip: Add roasted peanuts on top.

Nutritional Information Per Serving:
Calories 301 | Fat 16g |Sodium 189mg | Carbs 32g | Fiber 0.3g | Sugar 0.1g | Protein 28.2g

Chicken with Avocado Salsa

Prep Time: 15 minutes.

Cook Time: 42 minutes.

Serves: 2

Ingredients:

- 1 ½ pounds boneless chicken breasts

Marinade

- 2 garlic cloves, minced
- 3 tablespoons olive oil
- ¼ cup cilantro, chopped
- Juice of 1 lime
- ½ teaspoons salt
- ¼ teaspoons black pepper

Avocado Salsa

- 2 avocados, diced
- 2 small tomato, chopped
- ¼ cup red onion, chopped
- 1 jalapeno, deseeded and chopped
- 1/4 cup cilantro, chopped
- Juice of 1 lime
- Black pepper and salt to taste

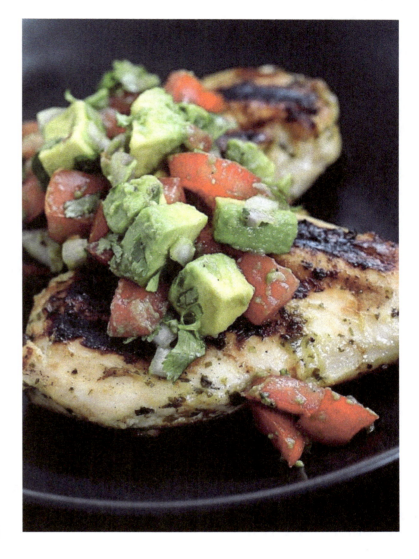

Preparation:

1. Mix all the marinade ingredients in a bowl.
2. Pound and flatten each chicken breast into ¼ inch thickness.
3. Add this chicken to the marinade, mix well, cover and refrigerate for 30 minutes.
4. Grill the chicken for 6 minutes per side in a preheated grill.
5. Serve the chicken with the avocado salsa.
6. Mix all the avocado salsa ingredients in a bowl.
7. Enjoy.

Serving Suggestion: Serve the chicken with cauliflower rice.

Variation Tip: Add dried herbs to the mixture for seasoning.

Nutritional Information Per Serving:

Calories 331 | Fat 20g |Sodium 941mg | Carbs 30g | Fiber 0.9g | Sugar 1.4g | Protein 24.6g

Chicken Piccata

Prep Time: 15 minutes.

Cook Time: 10 minutes.

Serves: 8

Ingredients:

- 8 boneless chicken breast halves
- 3 teaspoons olive oil
- 2 tablespoons butter
- 1/2 cup all-purpose flour
- 1/2 cup Parmesan cheese, grated
- 1/2 cup egg
- 1/2 teaspoon salt
- 2 tablespoons 1/4 cup dry white wine
- 1/4 cup parsley minced
- 1/8 teaspoon hot pepper sauce
- 5 tablespoons lemon juice
- 3 garlic cloves, minced

Preparation:

1. Pound and flatten each chicken piece.
2. Beat egg with hot pepper sauce, garlic, and 2 tablespoons lemon juice in a bowl.
3. Mix flour with salt, parsley, and Parmesan cheese in a bowl.
4. First coat the chicken with the flour mixture then dip in the egg mixture and coat again with the flour mixture.
5. Place the coated chicken a greased skillet and cook for 5 minutes per side.
6. Mix lemon juice, melted butter and remaining wine in a saucepan and boil.
7. Drizzle this sauce over the chicken.
8. Serve warm.

Serving Suggestion: Serve the chicken with a fresh crouton's salad.

Variation Tip: Add a drizzle of cheese on top.

Nutritional Information Per Serving:

Calories 300 | Fat 2g |Sodium 374mg | Carbs 30g | Fiber 6g | Sugar 3g | Protein 32g

Spinach Mushroom Chicken

Prep Time: 15 minutes.
Cook Time: 43 minutes.
Serves: 4

Ingredients:

- 6 ounces bag raw spinach leaves
- 2 ounces cream cheese
- 2 garlic cloves, minced
- 8 ounces baby bella mushrooms
- 2 teaspoons garlic powder
- 2 teaspoons salt
- 2 teaspoons ground thyme
- 4 chicken breasts
- 4 mozzarella cheese slices

Preparation:

1. At 400 degrees F, preheat your oven.
2. Season chicken with thyme, salt and 1 teaspoon garlic powder.
3. Place this chicken in a casserole dish and bake for 15 minutes in the oven.
4. Saute garlic in a skillet for 1 minute.
5. Stir in spinach and cook for 10 minutes.
6. Add cream cheese then mix well and remove from the heat.
7. Saute mushrooms with thyme, salt, and 1 teaspoon garlic powder in a skillet for 7 minutes.
8. Stir in cream cheese mixture and mix well.
9. Spread this mixture on top of the baked chicken.
10. Drizzle cheese on top and bake another 10 minutes.
11. Serve warm.

Serving Suggestion: Serve the chicken with toasted bread slices.

Variation Tip: Add butter sauce on top of the chicken before cooking.

Nutritional Information Per Serving:
Calories 419 | Fat 13g |Sodium 432mg | Carbs 9.1g | Fiber 3g | Sugar 1g | Protein 21g

Sesame Chicken

Prep Time: 15 minutes.
Cook Time: 20 minutes.
Serves: 2

Ingredients:

- 1 lb boneless chicken breasts, diced
- 1 large head of broccoli, chopped
- 2 red bell peppers, cut into chunks
- 1 cup snap peas
- Salt and black pepper, to taste
- Sesame seeds and green onions

Sauce:

- 1/4 cup soy sauce
- 1 tablespoon sweet chili sauce
- 2 tablespoons honey
- 2 garlic cloves
- 1 teaspoon fresh ginger

Preparation:

1. At 400 degrees F, preheat your oven.
2. Mix all the sauce ingredients in a saucepan and cook until it thickens.
3. Remove the sauce from the heat and allow the sauce to cool.
4. Spread the veggies and chicken in a greased baking sheet.
5. Drizzle sauce over the mixture and mix well.
6. Bake the mixture for 20 minutes in the oven.
7. Garnish with sesame seeds.
8. Serve warm.

Serving Suggestion: Serve the chicken with toasted bread on the side.

Variation Tip: Add some canned corn to the meal.

Nutritional Information Per Serving:
Calories 334 | Fat 16g |Sodium 462mg | Carbs 31g | Fiber 0.4g | Sugar 3g | Protein 25.3g

Beef, Pork, and Lamb

Green Lamb Curry

Prep Time: 15 minutes.
Cook Time: 2 hrs. 30 minutes.
Serves: 2

Ingredients:

- 2/3 lb. lean lamb, trimmed and diced
- 2½ tablespoons curry powder
- ½ teaspoons salt
- 1 tablespoon vegetable oil
- 2 onions, sliced
- 4 garlic cloves, chopped
- 1 tablespoon tomato purée
- ½ lb. fresh spinach
- Small bunch of coriander leaves, to serve
- Black pepper, to taste

Preparation:

1. Mix lamb meat with salt, black pepper and curry powder in a bowl.
2. Saute onions with oil in a skillet on medium heat until soft.
3. Stir in lamb and saute until brown.
4. Add garlic, tomato puree and water then cover and cook for 2 hours on medium heat.
5. Remove the lid and cook for 20 minutes.
6. Stir in spinach and cook for 3 minutes.
7. Garnish and serve warm.

Serving Suggestion: Serve the curry with white rice.

Variation Tip: Add some kale leaves instead of the spinach

Nutritional Information Per Serving:
Calories 305 | Fat 25g |Sodium 532mg | Carbs 2.3g | Fiber 0.4g | Sugar 2g | Protein 18.3g

Lamb Pea Curry

Prep Time: 15 minutes.
Cook Time: 22 minutes.
Serves: 2

Ingredients:

- 1 ¼ cups jasmine rice
- Cooking spray oil
- 14 ounces lean lamb medallions
- 5 teaspoons Thai green curry paste
- 1 red onion, sliced
- 14 ounces can creamy coconut evaporated milk
- 2 teaspoons fish sauce
- 1 ½ cups frozen peas
- 14 ounces mix carrot sticks, snow peas, amd broccoli florets

Preparation:

1. Sear the lamb with half of the curry paste and oil in a cooking pan for 2 minutes per side.
2. Cover this lamb and bake for 7 minutes at 400 degrees F.
3. Meanwhile, saute onion with remainig oil and curry paste in a skillet for 1 minute.
4. Stir in fish sauce and milk then cook for 5 minutes.
5. Add vegetables and cook for 5 minutes.
6. Slice the lamb and serve with veggies.
7. Enjoy.

Serving Suggestion: Serve the curry with toasted bread slices.

Variation Tip: Add crumbled feta cheese on top.

Nutritional Information Per Serving:
Calories 325 | Fat 16g |Sodium 431mg | Carbs 22g | Fiber 1.2g | Sugar 4g | Protein 23g

Lemon Lamb Chops

Prep Time: 15 minutes.

Cook Time: 18 minutes.

Serves: 8

Ingredients:

- Zest of 2 lemons
- 1 tablespoon oregano, chopped
- 1 ¼ teaspoons salt
- Black pepper to taste
- 8 lamb loin chops, trimmed
- 1/4 cup tahini
- ¼ cup nonfat yogurt
- ¼ cup seeded cucumber, diced
- ¼ cup lemon juice
- 2 garlic cloves, minced
- 1 tablespoon fresh parsley, chopped
- 3 tablespoons water
- 2 teaspoons olive oil

Preparation:

1. At 400 degrees F, preheat your ove,
2. Rub the lamb chops with black pepper ¾ teaspoons salt, oregano and lemon zest.
3. Cover and refrigerate these lamb chops for 1 hour.
4. Mix tahini with ½ teaspoons salt, parsley, garlic, lemon juice, cucumber and yogurt in a small bowl.
5. Sear lamb chops with oil in a skillet for 2 minutes per side.
6. Now bake them for 14 mintues in the oven.
7. Pour the tahini sauce on top.
8. Serve warm.

Serving Suggestion: Serve these chops with cauliflower rice.

Variation Tip: Add toasted croutons on top.

Nutritional Information Per Serving:

Calories 425 | Fat 14g |Sodium 411mg | Carbs 44g | Fiber 0.3g | Sugar 1g | Protein 28.3g

Braised Lamb Shanks

Prep Time: 15 minutes.
Cook Time: 2 hr. 30 minutes.
Serves: 4

Ingredients:

- 1 ½ pounds eggplant , peeled
- 4 (12-ounce) lamb shanks, trimmed
- 2 tablespoons ground sumac
- 1 ¼ teaspoons salt
- ½ teaspoon black pepper
- 2 tablespoons olive oil
- 1 green bell pepper, diced
- 1 small onion, diced
- 3 garlic cloves, minced
- 5 plum tomatoes, diced
- 1 cup water
- ½ cup parsley, chopped

Preparation:

1. Rub the lamb shanks with black pepper, salt and 1 tablespoon sumac.
2. Sear lamb with 1 tablespoon oil in a large Dutch oven for 5 minutes per side.
3. Transfer the lamb to a plate.
4. Add remaining 1 tablespoon oil, onion, minced garlic cloves, bell pepper and 1 tablespoon sumac.
5. Saute for 5 minutes then return the lamb to the pot.
6. Stir in tomatoes, water and eggplant then cover and cook on a simmer for 2 hours.
7. Remove the lid and cook for 10 minutes until the gravy thickens.
8. Garnish with parsley and serve warm.

Serving Suggestion: Serve the shanks with sweet potato salad.

Variation Tip: Add chopped green onion to the topping.

Nutritional Information Per Serving:
Calories 425 | Fat 15g |Sodium 345mg | Carbs 12.3g | Fiber 1.4g | Sugar 3g | Protein 23.3g

Lamb Cabbage Rolls

Prep Time: 15 minutes.
Cook Time: 1 hr. 10 minutes.
Serves: 8

Ingredients:

- ½ cup bulgur, cooked
- 1 large head Savoy cabbage
- 2 tablespoons olive oil
- 2 cups onion, chopped
- 1 cup leeks, chopped
- ¾ teaspoon salt
- ¾ teaspoon black pepper
- ½ teaspoon ground turmeric
- ¼ teaspoon ground ginger
- ¼ teaspoon ground allspice
- 1 pinch of ground cinnamon
- 12 ounces ground lamb
- ½ cup parsley, chopped
- 2 teaspoons fresh mint, chopped
- 1 large egg, beaten

- ½ cup white wine
- ½ cup chicken broth
- 2 teaspoons lemon zest, grated
- 3 tablespoons lemon juice

Preparation:

1. At 325 degrees F, preheat your oven.
2. Boil cabbage leaves in 2 ½ cups water in a cooking pan and drain.
3. Saute onion and leeks with oil in a skillet for 8 minutes.
4. Add cinnamon, allspice, ginger, turmeric, black pepper and salt then cook for 1 minute.
5. Transfer this mixture to a bowl and add bulgur.
6. Stir in lamb, parsley, mint and egg then mix well.
7. Spread the cabbage leaves o nthe working surface.
8. Divide the lamb filling at the center oeach leave.
9. Wrap the leaves around the filling and place the wrap in a baking dish.
10. Add lemon juice, lemon zest, broth and wine around the cabbage rolls.
11. Cover the dish with a foil sheet and bake for 1 hour in the oven.
12. Serve warm.

Serving Suggestion: Serve the rolls with roasted asparagus.

Variation Tip: Add a drizzle of parmesan cheese on top.

Nutritional Information Per Serving:
Calories 391 | Fat 5g |Sodium 88mg | Carbs 3g | Fiber 0g | Sugar 0g | Protein 27g

Pork With Caramelized Mushrooms

Prep Time: 15 minutes.
Cook Time: 20 minutes.
Serves: 2

Ingredients:

- 1 lb. lean ground pork
- 8 ounces mushrooms, sliced
- 1 small onion, sliced
- 1 tablespoon garlic, minced
- 1 tablespoon fresh ginger, grated
- 12 ounces bag whole green beans
- 2 tablespoons olive oil
- 1/4 cup water

SAUCE

- 2 tablespoons soy sauce
- 2 tablespoons mirin
- 1 tablespoon rice vinegar
- 2 teaspoons brown sugar
- 1 teaspoon sriracha
- 1 teaspoon dark sesame oil

Preparation:

1. Mix all the sauce ingredients in a small bowl.
2. Saute mushrooms with 1 tablespoon oil in a skillet until soft.
3. Stir in ground pork and saute until brown.
4. Add remaining oil, garlic, ginger, green beans and onion then saute for 2 minutes.
5. Stir in water and cook for another 2 minutes.
6. Pour in the prepared sauce and cook until the liquid is reduced to half.
7. Serve warm.

Serving Suggestion: Serve the pork with cauliflower rice.

Variation Tip: Add a layer of the boiled zucchini noodles to the stir fry.

Nutritional Information Per Serving:
Calories 376 | Fat 21g |Sodium 476mg | Carbs 12g | Fiber 3g | Sugar 4g | Protein 20g

Pepper Taco Bake

Prep Time: 15 minutes.

Cook Time: 30 minutes.

Serves: 4

Ingredients:

- 1 lb. lean ground beef
- 1 tablespoon Phoenix Sunrise Seasoning
- 1 cup vegetable salsa
- 1 ½ lbs fresh bell peppers, quartered
- 1/2 cup cheddar cheese, shredded
- 4 tablespoons sour cream

Preparation:

1. At 350 degrees F, preheat your oven.
2. Mix ground meat with salsa and seasoning in a large bowl.
3. Divide this mixture in the pepper halves and place these peppers in a baking dish.
4. Drizzle cheese on top and bake for 30 minutes in the oven.
5. Garnish with sour cream cheese and serve warm.

Serving Suggestion: Serve the bake with a fresh greens salad.

Variation Tip: Add chopped herbs on top.

Nutritional Information Per Serving:

Calories 487 | Fat 24g |Sodium 686mg | Carbs 17g | Fiber 1g | Sugar 1.2g | Protein 22g

Pan Seared Beef and Mushrooms

Prep Time: 15 minutes.
Cook Time: 17 minutes.
Serves: 4

Ingredients:

- 1 ½ lbs lean beef, cubed
- 1/2 tablespoon Dash of Desperation Seasoning
- Nonstick cooking spray
- 4 cups mushrooms, sliced
- 1 cup beef broth
- 1 ½ teaspoon Garlic Gusto Seasoning

Preparation:

1. Mix beef with seasoning and saute in a skillet with cooking spray for 7 minutes.
2. Add broth and rest of the ingredients and cook or 10 minutes with occasional stirring.
3. Serve warm.

Serving Suggestion: Serve the beef with sweet potato salad.

Variation Tip: Drizzle parmesan cheese on top before serving.

Nutritional Information Per Serving:
Calories 255 | Fat 12g |Sodium 66mg | Carbs 13g | Fiber 2g | Sugar 4g | Protein 22g

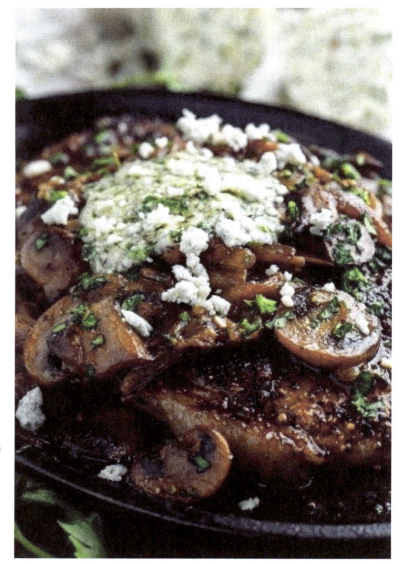

Sirloin with Horseradish Sauce

Prep Time: 15 minutes.

Cook Time: 14 minutes

Serves: 2

Ingredients:

- 1 ½ pounds sirloin steaks
- ½ tablesoon dash of desperation seasoning
- 6 tablespoons sour cream
- 3 tablespoons horseradish

Preparation:

1. At medium high heat heat, preheat your grill.
2. Season the steak with Dash seasoning and grill for 7 minutes per side.
3. Mix rest of the ingredients in a bowl.
4. Slice the grilled steak and pour the sauce over steak.
5. Serve warm.

Serving Suggestion: Serve the sirloin with fresh herbs on top.

Variation Tip: Add butter to the meat before serving.

Nutritional Information Per Serving:

Calories 405 | Fat 22.7g | Sodium 227mg | Carbs 26.1g | Fiber 1.4g | Sugar 0.9g | Protein 35.2g

Chipotle Pork Loin

Prep Time: 15 minutes.

Cook Time: 6 hours.

Serves: 4

Ingredients:

- 2 pounds boneless pork loin
- 1 tablespoon Garlic and Spring Onion Seasoning
- 1 tablespoon Cinnamon Chipotle Seasoning
- ¼ cup water

Preparation:

1. Add pork loin, water, seasoning and chipotle to a slow cooker.
2. Cover and cook for 6 hours on Low heat.
3. Serve warm.

Serving Suggestion: Serve the pork loin with sautéed carrots on the side.

Variation Tip: Drizzle parmesan cheese on top before serving.

Nutritional Information Per Serving:

Calories 345 | Fat 36g |Sodium 272mg | Carbs 41g | Fiber 0.2g | Sugar 0.1g | Protein 22.5g

Cauliflower Ground Beef Hash

Prep Time: 15 minutes.
Cook Time: 25 minutes.
Serves: 4

Ingredients:

- 16 ounces frozen cauliflower
- 1 lb. lean ground beef
- 2 cups cheddar cheese, shredded
- 1 teaspoon garlic powder
- Salt and black pepper to taste

Preparation:

1. Saute beef in a cooking pan until brown.
2. Stir in garlic, salt, black pepper and cauliflower then cook until soft.
3. Stir in cheddar cheese and cook until the cheese is melted.
4. Serve warm.

Serving Suggestion: Serve the beef hash with sautéed green beans and mashed sweet potatoes.

Variation Tip: Drizzle parmesan cheese on top before cooking.

Nutritional Information Per Serving:
Calories 395 | Fat 9.5g |Sodium 655mg | Carbs 13.4g | Fiber 0.4g | Sugar 0.4g | Protein 28.3g

Mojo Marinated Flank Steak

Prep Time: 15 minutes.

Cook Time: 10 minutes.

Serves: 4

Ingredients:

- 2 pounds flank steak
- 2 tablespoons fresh lime juice
- 1 tablespoon garlic Gusto seasoning
- 1 teaspoon ground cumin
- 1/3 cup beef broth
- 1 pinch Dash of Desperation Seasoning

Preparation:

1. Mix beef with remaining ingredients except dash seasoning, in a large bowl.
2. Cover the meat and refrigerate for 1 hour at least.
3. Preheat and grease a grill for cooking.
4. Remove the meat from the marinate and rub with the dash seasoning.
5. Grill the steak for 5 minutes per side.
6. Slice and serve warm.

Serving Suggestion: Serve the steaks with fresh green and mashed sweet potatoes.

Variation Tip: Add zucchini noodles on the side

Nutritional Information Per Serving:

Calories 301 | Fat 5g |Sodium 340mg | Carbs 24.7g | Fiber 1.2g | Sugar 1.3g | Protein 15.3g

Pork Loin with Tomatoes and Olives

Prep Time: 15 minutes.

Cook Time: 6 hours.

Serves: 4

Ingredients:

- 2 lbs pork tenderloin
- 1 cup chicken broth
- 2 teaspoons Garlic Gusto Seasoning
- 1/2 teaspoon Mediterranean Seasoning
- 10 green olives, sliced
- 1 tablespoon sun dried tomatoes, sliced

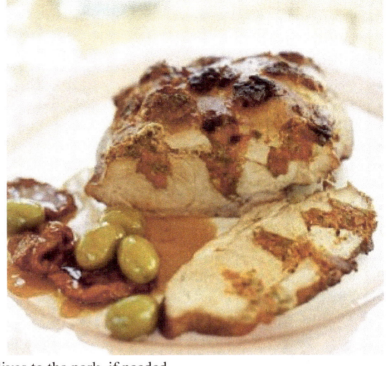

Preparation:

1. Add ork and all the ingredients to a crock pot and cover to a cook for 6 hours on Low heat.
2. Slice the meat and serve warm.

Serving Suggestion: Serve the pork with roasted green beans.

Variation Tip: Add sliced black kalamata olives to the pork, if needed.

Nutritional Information Per Serving:

Calories 448 | Fat 23g |Sodium 350mg | Carbs 18g | Fiber 6.3g | Sugar 1g | Protein 40.3g

Pork Tenderloins with Mushrooms

Prep Time: 15 minutes.
Cook Time: 32 minutes.
Serves: 6

Ingredients:

- Cooking spray
- 1 teaspoon dash seasoning
- 1 1/2 lbs pork tenderloin
- 6 cups portobello mushrooms, chopped
- 1/2 cup chicken broth
- 1 tablespoon garlic gusto
- Fresh parsley for garnish

Preparation:

1. At 400 degrees F, preheat your oven.
2. Rub the seasoning over the tenderloin.
3. Sear the tenderloin in a skillet, greased with cooking spray, for 3 minutes per side.
4. Trasnfer the seared pork to a plate.
5. Add rest of the ingredients to the same skillet and cook for 1 minute.
6. Return the pork tenderloin to the skillet and bake for 25 minutes.
7. Slice the pork and serve warm.

Serving Suggestion: Serve the pork with toasted bread slices.

Variation Tip: Replace mushrooms with chopped sweet potatoes.

Nutritional Information Per Serving:

Calories 309 | Fat 25g |Sodium 463mg | Cars 9.9g | Fiber 0.3g | Sugar 0.3g | Protein 28g

Herb Roasted Tenderloin

Prep Time: 15 minutes.
Cook Time: 60 minutes.
Serves: 8

Ingredients:

- 4 lbs pork tenderloin, lean
- 2 teaspoons black pepper
- 4 tablespoons parmesan cheese, grated
- 2 tablespoons fresh rosemary
- 1 tablespoon fresh thyme
- 1/2 teaspoon garlic, minced
- 1/2 teaspoon cumin
- 1/8 teaspoon salt
- 1 small onion, sliced
- 1/2 cup water

Preparation:

1. At 350 degrees, preheat your oven.
2. Mix cheese with spices in a bowl and rub over the pork.
3. Spread onion slices in a baking sheet and place the pork on top.
4. Add herbs on top and add ½ cup water around the pork.
5. Bake the pork for 1 hour in the preheated oven.
6. Serve warm.

Serving Suggestion: Serve the pork tenderloin with roasted green beans.

Variation Tip: Add paprika for more spice.

Nutritional Information Per Serving:

Calories 537 | Fat 20g |Sodium 719mg | Carbs 25.1g | Fiber 0.9g | Sugar 1.4g | Protein 37.8g

Fish and Seafood

Shrimp Salad

Prep Time: 15 minutes.
Cook Time: 17 minutes.
Serves: 2

Ingredients:

- 2 tablespoons olive oil
- 1/3 cup red onion, chopped
- 3 cups broccoli slaw
- 3 cups broccoli florets
- 1/2 teaspoon salt
- 2 garlic cloves, minced
- 1/2 pound shrimp, peeled and deveined
- 1 teaspoon lime juice
- Green onions, chopped, for garnish
- Cilantro, chopped
- Sriracha and red pepper flakes, for garnish

Sesame almond dressing:

- 2 tablespoons almond butter
- 2 tablespoons water
- 1 tablespoon sesame oil
- 1 tablespoon tamari
- 1 tablespoon maple syrup
- 1 teaspoon lime juice
- 1 teaspoon ginger, minced

- 1 clove minced garlic
- 1 teaspoon sriracha sauce
- 1/4 teaspoon black pepper

Preparation:

1. Mix all the sesame almond dressing in a bowl.
2. Saute onion with oil in a skillet for 5 minutes.
3. Stir in broccoli slaw and florest then saute for 7 minutes.
4. Add black pepper and salt then transfer to a plate.
5. Add minced garlic, shrimp, lime juice and more oil to the same skillet.
6. Saute for 5 minutes then transfer the shrimp to the broccoli.
7. Pour the sesame dressing on top and garnish with cilantro and green onions.
8. Serve warm.

Serving Suggestion: Serve the shrimp salad with cauliflower rice risotto.

Variation Tip: Add paprika for more spice.

Nutritional Information Per Serving:

Calories 212 | Fat 9g |Sodium 353mg | Carbs 8g | Fiber 3g | Sugar 4g | Protein 25g

Salmon Chowder

Prep Time: 15 minutes.
Cook Time: 20 minutes.
Serves: 6

Ingredients:

- 3 tablespoons olive oil
- 1 onion, diced
- 1 small fennel bulb, diced
- 1 cup celery, sliced
- 4 garlic cloves, chopped
- 1 teaspoon fennel seeds
- 1/2 teaspoon thyme
- 1/2 teaspoon smoked paprika
- 1/3 cup vermouth
- 3 cups fish stock
- 3/4 lb baby potatoes, sliced
- 1 teaspoon salt
- 1 bay leaf
- 1 lb salmon, skinless, diced
- 2 cups almond milk

Preparation:

1. lery, fennel, and onion witSaute ceh oil in a skillet for 6 minutes.
2. Stir in thyme, fennel seeds and garlic then saute for 2 minutes.
3. Add smoked paprika and vermouth then cook for 2 minutes.
4. Stir in salt, stock, bay, thyme, and potatoes then cook for 10 minutes on a simmer.
5. Stir in salmon bones, salt and milk then cook for 2 minutes.
6. Garnish with lemon wedges, fennel frongs and dill.
7. Serve warm.

Serving Suggestion: Serve the chowder with zucchini noodles.

Variation Tip: Add mixed chopped herbs and lemon zest to the chowder.

Nutritional Information Per Serving:

Calories 376 | Fat 17g |Sodium 1127mg | Carbs 24g | Fiber 1g | Sugar 3g | Protein 29g

Halibut With Zucchini Noodles

Prep Time: 15 minutes.

Cook Time: 17 minutes.

Serves: 8

Ingredients:

- 8 (10 ounces) halibut
- 1 garlic clove, smashed
- 2 tablespoons olive oil
- Salt and black pepper to taste

Noodles:

- 1 tablespoon olive oil
- 1 shallot, sliced
- 3 garlic cloves, chopped
- 16 ounces zucchini noodles
- Salt and black pepper to taste
- 2 teaspoons lemon zest
- ½ cup Italian parsley, chopped
- 1 tablespoon lemon juice

Preparation:

1. At 375 degrees F, preheat your oven.
2. Saute garlic with oil in a skillet over medium heat for 30 seconds.
3. Rub the black pepper and salt over the fish.
4. Sear this fish in the skillet for 6 minutes per side.
5. Transfer this fish to a plate and keep it aside.
6. Stir zucchini, black pepper and salt then saute for 4 minutes.
7. Stir in parsley, lemon zest and lemon juice.
8. Serve the zucchini noodles with fish on top.
9. Enjoy.

Serving Suggestion: Serve the noodles with fresh greens on the side.

Variation Tip: Roll the fish in breadcrumbs for a crispy touch.

Nutritional Information Per Serving:

Calories 457 | Fat 19g |Sodium 557mg | Carbs 19g | Fiber 1.8g | Sugar 1.2g | Protein 32.5g

Poached Mahi Mahi

Prep Time: 15 minutes.
Cook Time: 31 minutes.
Serves: 4

Ingredients:

- 4 (4-ounces) boneless mahi mahi fillets
- 1/4 teaspoon salt
- 1 cup olive oil
- 1 lb asparagus, trimmed
- 3 tablespoons olive oil
- 1 yellow onion, chopped
- 1/4 teaspoon black pepper
- 1 pinch red pepper glakes
- 10 green olives, pitted and chopped
- 1 small head garlic, minced
- 1 cup jarred roasted red peppers, chopped
- 2 tablespoons capers, drained, chopped
- 1/2 cup dry white wine
- 1/2 cup fresh basil, chopped
- 1 tablespoon fresh lemon juice
- Lemon wedges for serving

Preparation:

1. At 250 degrees F, preheat your oven.
2. Rub the fish with salt and keep it aside.
3. Add oil and fish to a skillet and sear for 3 minutes per side.
4. Bake this for 15 minutes then cover and keep it warm.
5. Saute onions with black pepper, pepper flakes and oil in a skillet for 4 minutes.
6. Stir in red pepper, capers, garlic and olives then cook for 2 minutes.
7. Add wine and cook the mixture for 3 minutes on a simmer.
8. Stir in asparagus tips and cook for 1 minute.
9. Add lemon juice, parsley and basil then over the fish.
10. Garnish with lemon wedges.
11. Serve warm.

Serving Suggestion: Serve the fish with cauliflower rice.

Variation Tip: Replace mahi mahi with codfish if needed.

Nutritional Information Per Serving:

Calories 392 | Fat 16g |Sodium 466mg | Carbs 3.9g | Fiber 0.9g | Sugar 0.6g | Protein 48g

Creamy Scallops

Prep Time: 15 minutes.
Cook Time: 9 minutes.
Serves: 3

Ingredients:

- 2 tablespoons olive oil
- 1 ¼ pounds scallops
- 2 tablespoons unsalted butter
- 5 garlic cloves, minced
- Salt and black pepper to taste
- 1/4 cup dry white wine
- 1 cup heavy cream
- 1 tablespoon lemon juice
- 1/4 cup parsley, chopped

Preparation:

1. Sear the scallops in a skillet with oil for 3 minutes per side.
2. Season them with black pepper and salt then transfer to a plate.
3. Saute garlic with 2 tablespoons butter in a skillet for 1 minute.
4. Stir in wine and cook for 2 minutes then add cream.
5. Cook this mixture until mixture thickens then add lemon juice.
6. Return the scallops to the skillet and garnish with parsley.
7. Serve warm.

Serving Suggestion: Serve the scallops with cauliflower salad.

Variation Tip: Add some cream cheese to the scallops.

Nutritional Information Per Serving:
Calories 316 | Fat 22g |Sodium 356mg | Carbs 7g | Fiber 2.4g | Sugar 5g | Protein 18g

Tuna Broccoli Mornay

Prep Time: 15 minutes.
Cook Time: 30 minutes.
Serves: 4

Ingredients:

- 1 x ½ lb. can Tuna in springwater, drained
- 3 oz. spiral pasta
- 1 head broccoli, florets
- 3 ½ ounce baby spinach leaves, washed
- 1 onion, diced
- 1 ounce butter
- 3 tablespoons flour
- Salt and black pepper, to taste
- 2 cups milk
- 1¼ cup grated cheese
- ¼ cup breadcrumbs

Preparation:

1. At 360 degrees F, preheat your oven.
2. Boil pasta as per the package's instructions then drain and keep it aside.
3. Saute onion with butter in a cooking pan until sfot.
4. Stir in flour and saute for 30 seconds.
5. Add milk, mix well and cook until the mixture thickens.
6. Add spinach and cook until the leaves are wilted.
7. Stir in 1 cup grated cheese, broccoli, tuna and black pepper.
8. Spread this mixture in a casserole dish and spread remaining cheese and breadcrumbs on top.
9. Bake for 25 minutes in the preheated oven.
10. Serve warm.

Serving Suggestion: Serve the mornay with sautéed vegetables.

Variation Tip: Add canned corn to the mornay.

Nutritional Information Per Serving:
Calories 258 | Fat 9g |Sodium 994mg | Carbs 1g | Fiber 0.4g | Sugar 3g | Protein 16g

Seared Scallops

Prep Time: 15 minutes.
Cook Time: 6 minutes.
Serves: 4

Ingredients:

- 1 lb. large scallops
- Salt, to taste
- Black pepper, , to taste
- 1 tablespoon olive oil
- 2 tablespoons butter
- 2 tablespoons parsley, chopped
- Lemon wedges, for serving

Preparation:

1. Season all the scallops with salt, balck pepper, and oil.
2. Melt butter and sear the scallops in a skillet for 3 minutes per side.
3. Drizzle parsley on top and garnish with lemon wedges.
4. Serve warm.

Serving Suggestion: Serve the scallops with lemon slices on top.

Variation Tip: Use white pepper for a change of flavor.

Nutritional Information Per Serving:

Calories 378 | Fat 21g |Sodium 146mg | Carbs 7.1g | Fiber 0.1g | Sugar 0.4g | Protein 23g

Thai Green Curry

Prep Time: 15 minutes.
Cook Time: 10 minutes.
Serves: 2

Ingredients:

- Fish
- 2 cod fillets
- 2 halibut fillets
- 2 snapper fillets
- 1 lemon
- 2 cups coconut milk
- 3 ounces baby spinach
- 2 ounces carrots, shredded

Preparation:

1. Add coconut milk and rest of the ingredients to a cooking pot.
2. Cook this mixture for 10 minutes on medium heat.
3. Serve warm.

Serving Suggestion: Serve the curry with white rice.

Variation Tip: Drizzle cheese on top for a rich taste.

Nutritional Information Per Serving:

Calories 351 | Fat 4g |Sodium 236mg | Carbs 19.1g | Fiber 0.3g | Sugar 0.1g | Protein 36g

Grilled salmon with Avocado Salsa

Prep Time: 15 minutes.
Cook Time: 10 minutes.
Serves: 4

Ingredients:

- 2 lbs. salmon, cut into 4 fillets
- 1 tablespoon of olive oil
- 1 teaspoon of salt
- 1 teaspoon of cumin
- 1 teaspoon of paprika
- 1 teaspoon of onion
- 1/2 teaspoon chili spices
- 1 teaspoon black pepper

Salsa:

- 1 avocado chopped
- ½ small red onion, sliced
- Juice of 2 limes
- 1 tablespoon of fresh coriander
- Salt, to taste

Preparation:

1. Mix all the spices in a bowl and rub over the salmon fillets along with olive oil.
2. Grill the salmon fillet for 5 minutes per side in a preheated grill.
3. Chopped avocados with rest of the ingredients in a bowl.
4. Serve the grilled fish with avocado mash on top.
5. Enjoy.

Serving Suggestion: Serve the salmon with sweet potato salad.

Variation Tip: Add some chopped bell pepper to the meal.

Nutritional Information Per Serving:

Calories 378 | Fat 7g |Sodium 316mg | Carbs 16.2g | Fiber 0.3g | Sugar 0.3g | Protein 26g

Lemon Garlic Cod with Tomatoes

Prep Time: 15 minutes.

Cook Time: 45 minutes.

Serves: 2

Ingredients:

- 1 ½ pounds cod
- 2 pints cherry tomatoes
- 2 tablespoons olive oil
- 1 teaspoon salt
- 3 garlic cloves, sliced
- 1 tablespoon fresh sage, chopped
- 2 lemons, sliced
- 2 tablespoons capers, for garnish

Preparation:

1. At 325 degrees F, preheat your oven.
2. Place cod in a greased 9x13 inches baking dish.
3. Add tomatoes, olive oil, garlic, sage, lemon and salt on top of the cod.
4. Bake the cod for 45 minutes in the oven.
5. Garnish with capers then serve warm.

Serving Suggestion: Serve the cod with roasted broccoli florets.

Variation Tip: Drizzle lemon zest on top before cooking.

Nutritional Information Per Serving:

Calories 415 | Fat 15g |Sodium 634mg | Carbs 14.3g | Fiber 1.4g | Sugar 1g | Protein 23.3g

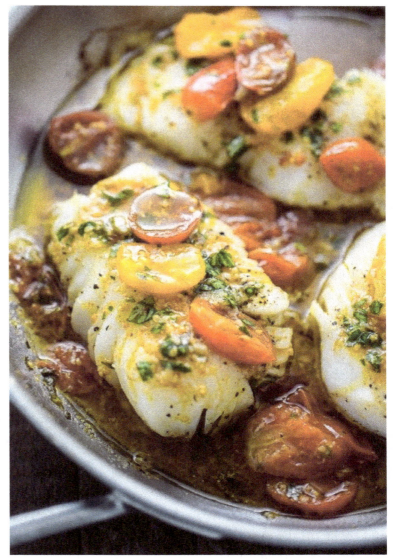

Shrimp Pineapple

Prep Time: 15 minutes.

Cook Time: 15 minutes.

Serves: 4

Ingredients:

- 1 cup pineapple, chopped
- 1lb raw jumbo shrimp
- 1 ½ tablespoons arrowroot starch
- 2 tablespoons avocado oil

Sauce

- 1 tablespoon ginger, minced
- 2/3 cup pineapple juice
- 1 tablespoon garlic, minced
- 3 tablespoon sriracha
- 1 tablespoon soy sauce
- 2 teaspoons arrowroot starch
- 1 tablespoon garlic, minced
- 1 tablespoon honey
- 1/3 cup bell pepper, diced

Garnish

- Fresh green onion
- Sesame seeds
- Fresh limen

Preparation:

1. Mix all the sauce ingredients in a bowl and keep it aside.
2. Toss shrimp with arrowroot in a bowl and shake off the excess.
3. Set a skillet with olive oil over medium heat.
4. Stir in pineapple chunks and cook for 5 minutes.
5. Transfer to a plate and keep them aside.
6. Saute shrimp with avocado oil in the same skillet for 8 minutes.
7. Stir in bell peppers then saute for 1 minute.
8. Add prepared sauce and mix well.
9. Stir in pineapple juice and chunks.
10. Cook for 30 seconds then serve warm.

Serving Suggestion: Serve these shrimp with boiled white rice.

Variation Tip: Add garlic salt to the seasoning for more taste.

Nutritional Information Per Serving:

Calories 251 | Fat 17g |Sodium 723mg | Carbs 21g | Fiber 2.5g | Sugar 2g | Protein 7.3g

Fish Green Curry

Prep Time: 15 minutes.

Cook Time: 13 minutes.

Serves: 4

Ingredients:

- 1 (15-ounce can) coconut milk
- 2 tablespoons green curry paste
- 1 (1-inch) nub fresh ginger, peeled and grated
- 2 tablespoons lime juice
- 2 tablespoons fish sauce
- 1 crown broccoli, chopped
- 2 cups green beans, chopped
- 1 zucchini squash, chopped
- 2 pounds white fish
- Salt, to taste

Serving

- Coconut milk yogurt
- Chives

Preparation:

1. Add coconut milk, lime juice, fish sauce, ginger, and curry paste to a cooking pot and cook to a boil.
2. Stir in green beans and broccoli and cook for 3 minutes.
3. Stir fish and zucchnini, cover and cook for 10 minutes.
4. Serve warm.

Serving Suggestion: Serve the fish curry with cauliflower rice.

Variation Tip: Add olives or sliced mushrooms to the fish.

Nutritional Information Per Serving:

Calories 246 | Fat 15g |Sodium 220mg | Carbs 40.3g | Fiber 2.4g | Sugar 1.2g | Protein 12.4g

Vegetables and Sides

Vegan Meatballs

Prep Time: 20 minutes.
Cook Time: 48 minutes.
Serves: 4

Ingredients:

- 1 cup cooked quinoa
- 1 (15-ounce) can black beans
- 2 tablespoons water
- 3 garlic cloves, minced
- 1/2 cup shallot, diced
- 1/4 teaspoon salt
- 2 1/2 teaspoon fresh oregano
- 1/2 teaspoon red pepper flake
- 1/2 teaspoon fennel seeds
- 1/2 cup vegan parmesan cheese, shredded
- 2 tablespoons tomato paste
- 3 tablespoons fresh basil, chopped
- 2 tablespoons worcestershire sauce

Preparation:

1. At 350 degrees F, preheat your oven.
2. Spread the beans in a baking sheet and bake for 15 minutes.
3. Meanwhile, saute garlic, shallots and water to a skillet for 3 minutes.
4. Transfer to the food processor along with fennel, red pepper flakes, baked beans, oregano and salt.
5. Blend these ingredients just until incorporated.
6. Stir in quinoa, and rest of the ingredients then mix evenly.
7. Make golf-ball sized meatballs out of this mixture.
8. Spread these meatballs in a grease baking sheet and bake for 20-30 minutes until brown.
9. Flip the meatballs once cooked half way through.
10. Serve warm.

Serving Suggestion: Serve the meatballs with pita bread and chili sauce.

Variation Tip: Add chopped mushrooms to the batter as well.

Nutritional Information Per Serving:
Calories 338 | Fat 24g |Sodium 620mg | Carbs 58.3g | Fiber 2.4g | Sugar 1.2g | Protein 5.4g

Minestrone Soup

Prep Time: 15 minutes.

Cook Time: 40 minutes.

Serves: 6

Ingredients:

- 1 yellow onion, diced
- 3 garlic cloves, minced
- 1 carrot peeled and diced
- 4 celery stalks, diced
- 4 cups vegetable broth
- 1 (15-ounces) can of tomato juice
- 1 (15-ounces) can of diced tomatoes
- 8 ounces elbow pasta
- 1 (15ounces) can of red kidney beans rinsed and drained
- 1 (15ounces) can of white beans
- 2 handfuls baby spinach, chopped
- 1 teaspoon coriander
- 1 teaspoon oregano
- 1 teaspoon black pepper
- 1 teaspoon basil
- 1 teaspoon paprika
- Salt to taste
- Chopped parsley for garnish

Preparation:

1. Add carrot, garlic, celery, onion and vegetable broth in a cooking pot and cook for 20 minutes on a simmer.
2. Stir in rest of the ingredients and cook for 20 minutes.
3. Garnish with parsley.
4. Serve warm.

Serving Suggestion: Serve the soup with avocado salad.

Variation Tip: Add chopped mushrooms to the soup as well.

Nutritional Information Per Serving:

Calories 393 | Fat 3g |Sodium 510mg | Carbs 12g | Fiber 3g | Sugar 4g | Protein 4g

Tofu Fried Rice

Prep Time: 10 minutes.

Cook Time: 13 minutes.

Serves: 4

Ingredients:

- 1 package baked tofu
- 4 cup cauliflower rice
- 1 cup frozen peas
- 1 cup carrots, shredded
- 1 teaspoon onion powder
- 1 teaspoon garlic powder
- 1/2 cup soy sauce
- 1/4 cup scallions, chopped
- Salt and black pepper to taste

Preparation:

1. Saue tofu with peas, carrots, garlic powder, soy sauce, scallions, black pepper and salt in a cooking pan for 10 minutes.
2. Stir in cauliflower rice and mix well.
3. Cover and cook for 3 minutes on medium heat.
4. Serve warm.

Serving Suggestion: Serve the rice with kale salad.

Variation Tip: Add boiled couscous to the mixture.

Nutritional Information Per Serving:

Calories 378 | Fat 3.8g |Sodium 620mg | Carbs 13.3g | Fiber 2.4g | Sugar 1.2g | Protein 5.4g

Rice and Beans

Prep Time: 15 minutes.
Cook Time: 22 minutes.
Serves: 4

Ingredients:

- 1 cup dry brown rice
- 1 ½ cup water
- 1 can of black beans
- 1 teaspoon paprika
- 1 teaspoon garlic powder
- 1 teaspoon oregano
- 1 teaspoon cumin
- 1 teaspoon onion powder

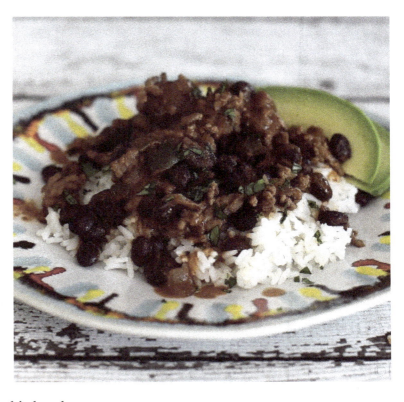

Preparation:

1. At 350 degrees F, preheat your oven.
2. Add water and rice to the Instant Pot's insert.
3. Set a trivet over the rice and place a baking dish on top.
4. Add beans and rest of the ingreidnets to this bowl.
5. Cover and seal the lid and cook for 22 minutes at Low pressure.
6. Once done, release all the pressure and remove the lid.
7. Mix the beans and transfer to a serving plate.
8. Serve the beans with the rice.
9. Enjoy.

Serving Suggestion: Serve the beans with the spinach salad.

Variation Tip: Add crispy fried onion on top for better taste.

Nutritional Information Per Serving:

Calories 304 | Fat 31g |Sodium 834mg | Carbs 21.4g | Fiber 0.2g | Sugar 0.3g | Protein 4.6g

Corn Chowder

Prep Time: 15 minutes.
Cook Time: 28 minutes.
Serves: 8

Ingredients:

- 4 cups vegetable broth
- 8 cups corn
- 1 whole yellow onion, diced
- 1 tablespoon chili powder
- 1 teaspoon salt
- 4 cups water
- 1/4 cup nutritional yeast
- 1/4 lime juiced
- 1/4 cup cilantro

Preparation:

1. Add vegetable broth, onion, corn and chili powder to a cooking pot.
2. Cook for 8 minutes with occasional stirring.
3. Remove 1/3 of this cooking mixture and keep it aside.
4. Add water to the rest and cook for 20 minutes on a simmer.
5. Puree the cooked corn soup until smooth.
6. Stir in lime juice, yeast, and remaining corn mixture.
7. Serve warm with cilantro on top.
8. Enjoy.

Serving Suggestion: Serve the chowder with cauliflower salad.

Variation Tip: Top the chowder cheddar cheese with before serving.

Nutritional Information Per Serving:

Calories 341 | Fat 24g |Sodium 547mg | Carbs 36.4g | Fiber 1.2g | Sugar 1g | Protein 10.3g

Asian Slaw

Prep Time: 15 minutes.

Cook Time: 0 minutes.

Serves: 4

Ingredients:

Salad:

- 2 cups green cabbage, shredded
- 1/2 cup carrots, shredded
- 1/2 cup cilantro, chopped
- 1/2 cup bell peppers, sliced
- 1/2 cup peanuts, crushed
- Avocado slices

Dressing:

- 2 tablespoons peanut butter
- 1 teaspoon agave syrup
- 1 tablespoon soy sauce
- 1 teaspoon white wine vinegar
- 1 teaspoon lime juice
- 1 tablespoon water
- Salt and black black pepper to taste

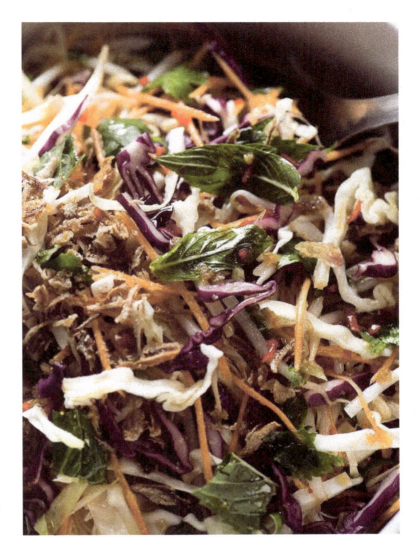

Preparation:

1. First, mix all the dressing ingredients in a salad bowl.
2. Stir in rest of the slaw ingredients and mix well.
3. Serve.

Serving Suggestion: Serve the slaw with turkey burgers.

Variation Tip: Add some edamame beans to the bowl.

Nutritional Information Per Serving:

Calories 318 | Fat 15.7g |Sodium 124mg | Carbs 27g | Fiber 0.1g | Sugar 0.3g | Protein 4.9g

Spinach Alfredo Soup

Prep Time: 15 minutes.

Cook Time: 23 minutes.

Serves: 6

Ingredients:

- 2 cups cauliflower florets
- 1/2 teaspoon garlic, minced
- 1 teaspoon olive oil
- ½ cup cottage cheese
- 9 ounces shredded cheese
- 6 wedges Light Laughing Cow cheese
- ½ teaspoon salt
- ¼ teaspoon black pepper
- 1 cup cashew milk
- 26 ounces frozen Spinach
- 3 tablespoon Parmesan cheese, shredded
- 18 ounces yogurt

Preparation:

1. Boil cauliflower in a cooking pan filled with water for 10 minutes.
2. Traansfer the cauliflower florets to a blender along with 1 cup cooking liquid.
3. Puree this mixture and keep it aside.
4. Saute garlic with olive oil in a suitable pan for 3 minutes.
5. Transfer to the cauliflower and add all these cheese, black pepper, milk and salt.
6. Blend these ingredients together until smooth.
7. Return the mixture to the saucepan and add one more cup of cooking liquid.
8. Cook the soup to a boil then add spinach and cook for 10 minutes.
9. Serve warm.

Serving Suggestion: Serve the soup with cauliflower rice.

Variation Tip: Add broccoli florets to the soup as well.

Nutritional Information Per Serving:

Calories 314 | Fat 2.2g |Sodium 276mg | Carbs 27.7g | Fiber 0.9g | Sugar 1.4g | Protein 8.8g

Artichoke Stuffed Mushroom

Prep Time: 15 minutes.

Cook Time: 20 minutes.

Serves: 8

Ingredients:

- 8 (1/2 ounces) Portobello Mushroom, caps

Filling ingredients:

- 1/4 cup alfredo sauce
- 2 wedges light laughing cow cheese
- 1 teaspoon garlic, minced
- 1 egg
- 4 ounces cheese, shredded
- 1-1/2 cup light cottage cheese
- 1/2 cup hearts of palm, diced
- 1 cup spinach, shredded
- 4 tablespoons parmesan, shredded

Preparation:

1. Mix all the filling ingredients in a suitable bowl.
2. Divide this mixture in the mushroom caps.
3. Place these stuffed caps in a greased baking sheet.
4. Bake them for 20 minutes at 350 degrees F in the oven.
5. Serve warm.

Serving Suggestion: Serve the mushrooms with kale salad.

Variation Tip: Add lemon zest and lemon juice for better taste.

Nutritional Information Per Serving:

Calories 324 | Fat 5g |Sodium 432mg | Carbs 13.1g | Fiber 0.3g | Sugar 1g | Protein 5.7g

Asparagus With Garlic

Prep Time: 15 minutes.
Cook Time: 45 minutes.
Serves: 4

Ingredients:

- 1 lb. thick asparagus spears, trimmed and chopped
- ½ cup garlic cloves, peeled and chopped
- 3 tablespoons olive oil
- Salt and black pepper, to taste

Preparation:

1. Mix asparagus with garlic, olive oil, black pepper and salt in a bowl.
2. Cover and marinate for 30 minutes.
3. Meanwhile, at 450 degrees F, preheat your oven.
4. Spread the asparagus in a baking sheet.
5. Roast them for 15 minutes in the preheated oven.
6. Serve warm.

Serving Suggestion: Serve the asparagus with toasted bread slices.

Variation Tip: Add boiled zucchini pasta to the mixture.

Nutritional Information Per Serving:

Calories 136 | Fat 10g |Sodium 249mg | Carbs 8g | Fiber 2g | Sugar 3g | Protein 4g

Avocado Tomato Salad

Prep Time: 15 minutes.
Cook Time: 14 minutes.
Serves: 2

Ingredients:

- 2 ripe avocados
- 2 ripe beefsteak tomatoes
- 2 tablespoons lemon juice
- 3 tablespoons cilantro, chopped
- Salt and black pepper to taste

Preparation:

1. Peel the avocados, remove their pits and cut into cubes.
2. Transfer the avocados to a salad bowl.
3. Stir in toamtoes, lemon juice, cilantro, black pepper and salt.
4. Mix well and serve fresh.

Serving Suggestion: Serve the salad with grilled salmon.

Variation Tip: Add canned corn to the salad.

Nutritional Information Per Serving:
Calories 151 | Fat 9g |Sodium 412mg | Carbs 43g | Fiber 0.3g | Sugar 1g | Protein 3g

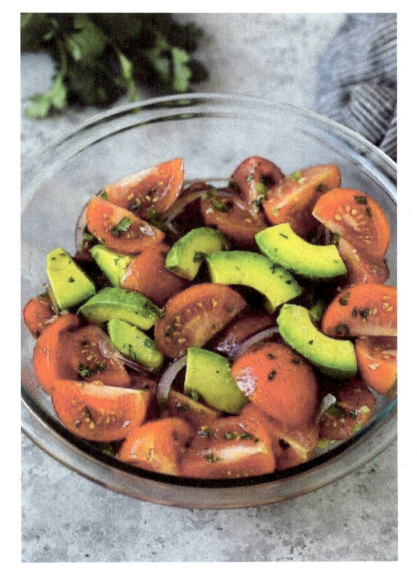

Dessert Recipes

Chia Seed Pudding

Prep Time: 15 minutes.
Cook Time: 0 minute.
Serves: 2

Ingredients:

- 2 cups almond milk
- 1/2 cup chia seeds
- 1/4 cup almond butter
- 1/4 cup cocoa powder unsweetened
- 4 dates large, pitted and chopped
- 1 teaspoon pure vanilla extract

Preparation:

1. Blend all the pudding ingredients in a bowl.
2. Cover and refrigerate this pudding for 4 hours.
3. Serve.

Serving Suggestion: Serve the pudding with goji berries on top.

Variation Tip: Add white chocolate syrup on top.

Nutritional Information Per Serving:

Calories 361 | Fat 10g |Sodium 218mg | Carbs 56g | Fiber 10g | Sugar 30g | Protein 4g

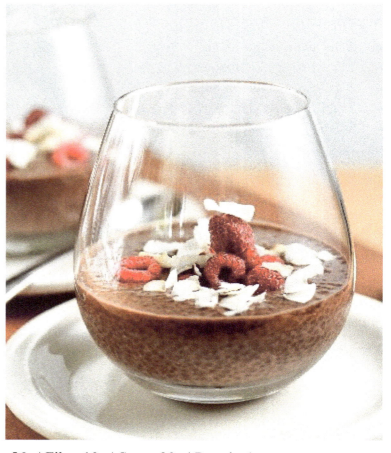

Strawberry Ice Cream

Prep Time: 10 minutes.

Cook Time: 0 minutes.

Serves: 6

Ingredients:

- 16 ounce strawberries, frozen
- 3/4 cup Greek yogurt plain
- 2 tablespoons balsamic vinegar
- 2 tablespoons honey

Preparation:

1. Blend all the ingredients for ice cream in a blender until smooth.
2. Divide the mixture in the ice-cream molds.
3. Freeze the ice cream for 4 hours.
4. Serve.

Serving Suggestion: Serve the ice cream with fresh berries on top.

Variation Tip: Add strawberry preserves on top of the ice cream.

Nutritional Information Per Serving:

Calories 118 | Fat 20g |Sodium 192mg | Carbs 23.7g | Fiber 0.9g | Sugar 19g | Protein 5.2g

Strawberry Yogurt

Prep Time: 5 minutes.

Cook Time: 0 minutes.

Serves: 2

Ingredients:

Spices

- 1 cup Greek yogurt plain
- 3/4 cup strawberry fruit spread

Preparation:

1. Blend yogurt with strawberries in a blender.
2. Serve.

Serving Suggestion: Serve the yogurt with berries on top.

Variation Tip: Add chopped pecans to the yogurt as well.

Nutritional Information Per Serving:

Calories 248 | Fat 16g |Sodium 95mg | Carbs 38.4g | Fiber 0.3g | Sugar 10g | Protein 14.1g

Banana Pops

Prep Time: 15 minutes.

Cook Time: 0 minutes.

Serves: 2

Ingredients:

- 3 bananas
- 3 tablespoons cacao powder raw
- 2 liquid stevia drops
- 3 ounces water
- 1/4 cup cacao nibs raw
- 1/4 cup goji berries raw

Preparation:

1. Insert a stick into each banana.
2. Place these bananas in the freezer for 30 minutes.
3. Mash the remaining banana with stevia, water and cacao powder in a bowl.
4. Dip the bananas on the stick in the cacao mmixture.
5. Coat them with cacao nibs and gji berries.
6. Serve.

Serving Suggestion: Serve the pops with chocolate or apple sauce.

Variation Tip: Dip the bananas in white chocolate syrup.

Nutritional Information Per Serving:

Calories 117 | Fat 12g |Sodium 79mg | Carbs 24.8g | Fiber 1.1g | Sugar 18g | Protein 5g

Strawberry Cheesecake

Prep Time: 15 minutes.

Cook Time: 0 minutes.

Serves: 6

Ingredients:

- 1/2 cup cream cheese
- 2 tablespoons coconut palm sugar
- 1/2 cup Greek yogurt
- 2 teaspoons lemon juice, squeezed
- 1/4 cup strawberry preserves
- 1 cup strawberries diced
- 1/3 cup almonds whole
- 4 dates

Preparation:

1. Beat cream cheese with lemon juice, yogurt, and sugar in a blender for 3 minutes.
2. Mix strawberries with preserves in a small bowl.
3. Grind the almonds with dates in a food processor.
4. Divide the almond mixture in a muffin tray and press it.
5. Add cheesecake batter on top and divide the strawberry mixture on top.
6. Refirgerate these mini cheese cakes for 1 hour.
7. Serve.

Serving Suggestion: Serve the cheese cakes with creamy frosting on top.

Variation Tip: Add chopped pecans or walnuts to the batter.

Nutritional Information Per Serving:

Calories 195 | Fat 3g | Sodium 355mg | Carbs 20g | Fiber 1g | Sugar 25g | Protein 1g

Coffee Cake Muffins

Prep Time: 15 minutes.

Cook Time: 15 minutes.

Serves: 4

Ingredients:

- 1 packet medifast cappuccino
- 1 packet medifast chocolate chip pancakes
- 1 packet of stevia
- 1 tablespoon egg, beaten
- 1/4 teaspoon baking powder
- 1/4 cup water

Preparation:

1. Mix cappuccino fueling and rest of the ingredients in a bowl until smooth.
2. Divide the mixture into the muffin tray.
3. Bake the muffins for 15 minutes in the oven at 350 degrees F.
4. Allow the muffins to cool and serve.

Serving Suggestion: Serve the muffins with chopped nuts on top.

Variation Tip: Add dried raisins to the muffins.

Nutritional Information Per Serving:

Calories 203 | Fat 8.9g |Sodium 340mg | Carbs 24.7g | Fiber 1.2g | Sugar 11.3g | Protein 5.3g

Peanut Butter Balls

Prep Time: 15 minutes.
Cook Time: 0 minutes.
Serves: 4

Ingredients:

- 1 Medifast chocolate pudding
- 1 Medifast chocolate shake
- 4 tablespoons powdered peanut butter
- 2 tablespoons water
- 1/4 cup unsweetened almond milk

Preparation:

1. Mix chocolate pudding and all the ingredients in a bowl.
2. Make 8 fudge balls out of this mixture.
3. Place the fudge balls in a baking sheet and refrigerate for 4 hours.
4. Serve.

Serving Suggestion: Serve the balls with chopped nuts on top.

Variation Tip: Add vanilla extracts to the dessert.

Nutritional Information Per Serving:

Calories 153 | Fat 1g |Sodium 8mg | Carbs 66g | Fiber 0.8g | Sugar 56g | Protein 1g

Brownie in a Tray

Prep Time: 15 minutes.
Cook Time: 1 minutes.
Serves: 4

Ingredients:

- 1 Medifast Brownie Mix
- 3 tablespoons water
- 1 wedge cream cheese
- 2 tablespoons Peanut butter powder
- 1 tablespoon water

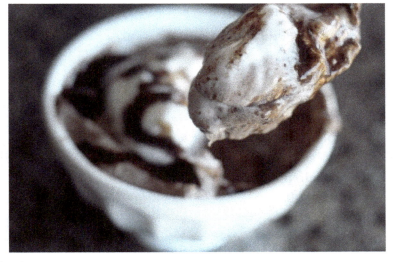

Preparation:

1. Blend brownie mix with 3 tbs water in a shallow bowl.
2. Heat this mixture in the microwave for 1 minutes.
3. Slice the cream cheese slices and place on top of the brownie.
4. Blend peanut butter powder with 1 tablespoon water in a bowl.
5. Pour this mixture over the brownie.
6. Serve.

Serving Suggestion: Serve the brownie with chocolate syrup or berries on top.

Variation Tip: Add crushed walnuts or pecans to the brownie.

Nutritional Information Per Serving:

Calories 198 | Fat 14g |Sodium 272mg | Carbs 34g | Fiber 1g | Sugar 9.3g | Protein 1.3g

Dark Chocolate Mousse

Prep Time: 10 minutes.
Cook Time: 0 minutes.
Serves: 2

Ingredients:

- 2 ripe avocados, peeled and pitted
- ½ cup dark cocoa powder
- 1 tablespoon vanilla extract
- ¼ cup stevia powder
- ¼ cup almond milk
- 1 pinch salt

Preparation:

1. Blend all avocados with rest of the ingredients in a blender until smooth.
2. Cover and refrigerate the mousse for 1 hour.
3. Garnish and serve.

Serving Suggestion: Serve the mousse with chocolate sauce on top.

Variation Tip: Add crushed nuts or coconut flakes.

Nutritional Information Per Serving:
Calories 159 | Fat 3g |Sodium 277mg | Carbs 21g | Fiber 1g | Sugar 9g | Protein 2g

Banana Pudding

Prep Time: 10 minutes.
Cook Time: 15 minutes.
Serves: 4

Ingredients:
Cookie layer:
- 2 tablespoons butter softened
- 1 teaspoon vanilla extract
- 1 egg
- 1/2 cup almond flour
- 1 teaspoon baking powder
- 1/4 cup erythritol

Pudding layer:
- 2 cups heavy whipping cream
- 1 cup almond milk
- 2 teaspoons vanilla extract
- 6 egg yolks
- 1/2 cup erythritol
- 1 medium banana, sliced

Whipped cream layer:
- 1/2 cup heavy whipping cream
- 1 teaspoon vanilla extract
- 1/4 cup erythritol
- 1/4 teaspoon xanthan gum

Preparation:
1. At 350 degrees F, preheat your oven.
2. Layer a baking sheet with parchment paper.
3. Mix butter with egg and vanilla in a bowl.
4. Stir in baking powder, almond flour and erythritol then mix well.
5. Spread this mixture in a 8x16 inches baking sheet.
6. Bake this batter for 15 minutes until golden brown.
7. Meanwhile, mix all the pudding ingredients in a saucepan and cook until the pudding thickens.
8. Spread the pudding over the baked cookie layer.
9. Beat all the cream layer ingredients in a bowl until fluffy.
10. Spread this mixture over the pudding layer.
11. Cover and refrigerate for 1 hour.
12. Slice and serve.

Serving Suggestion: Serve the pudding cups with peanut butter frosting on top.
Variation Tip: Add chocolate chips or a teaspoon of crushed nuts to the batter for the change of flavor.
Nutritional Information Per Serving:
Calories 268 | Fat 14g |Sodium 122mg | Carbs 23.3g | Fiber 1.2g | Sugar 12g | Protein 6g

5 &1 Meal Plan

Week 1

Day 1:

Fueling Hacks:

Cranberry Sweet Potato Muffins

Baked Kale Chips

Grilled Buffalo Shrimp

Buckwheat Crepes

Oatmeal Pancakes

Lean and Green Meal:

Seared Scallops

Day 2:

Fueling Hacks:

Celery Salad

Yogurt Trail Mix Bars

Quinoa Pudding

Curried Tuna Salad

Tuna Quinoa Cakes

Lean and Green Meal:

Turkey Taco Soup

Day 3:

Fueling Hacks:

Taco Salad

Cranberry Sweet Potato Muffins

Quinoa Bars

Yogurt Trail Mix Bars

Oatmeal Pancakes

Lean and Green Meal:

Creamy Scallops

Day 4:

Fueling Hacks:

Buckwheat Crepes

Baked Kale Chips

Grilled Buffalo Shrimp

Celery Salad

Curried Tuna Salad

Tuna Quinoa Cakes

Lean and Green Meal:

Mojo Marinated Flank Steak

Day 5:

Fueling Hacks:

Quinoa Pudding

Yogurt Trail Mix Bars

Curried Tuna Salad

Tuna Quinoa Cakes

Lean and Green Meal:

Poached Mahi Mahi

Day 6:

Fueling Hacks:

Celery Salad

Baked Kale Chips

Grilled Buffalo Shrimp

Curried Tuna Salad

Cranberry Sweet Potato Muffins

Lean and Green Meal:

Pork Loin with Tomatoes and Olives

Day 7:

Fueling Hacks:

Cranberry Sweet Potato Muffins

Quinoa Bars

Tuna Quinoa Cakes

Buckwheat Crepes

Yogurt Trail Mix Bars

Lean and Green Meal:

Cauliflower Ground Beef Hash

Week 2

Day 1:

Fueling Hacks:

Quinoa Pudding

Cranberry Sweet Potato Muffins

Baked Kale Chips

Grilled Buffalo Shrimp

Oatmeal Pancakes

Lean and Green Meal:

Seared Scallops

Day 2:

Fueling Hacks:

Quinoa Pudding

Celery Salad

Taco Salad

Yogurt Trail Mix Bars

Tuna Quinoa Cakes

Lean and Green Meal:

Turkey Taco Soup

Day 3:

Fueling Hacks:

Curried Tuna Salad

Cranberry Sweet Potato Muffins

Quinoa Bars

Buckwheat Crepes

Celery Salad

Lean and Green Meal:

Creamy Scallops

Day 4:

Fueling Hacks:

Oatmeal Pancakes

Baked Kale Chips

Grilled Buffalo Shrimp

Curried Tuna Salad

Celery Salad

Lean and Green Meal:

Mojo Marinated Flank Steak

Day 5:

Fueling Hacks:

Tuna Quinoa Cakes

Taco Salad

Yogurt Trail Mix Bars

Curried Tuna Salad

Tuna Quinoa Cakes

Lean and Green Meal:

Poached Mahi Mahi

Day 6:

Fueling Hacks:

Yogurt Trail Mix Bars

Celery Salad

Taco Salad

Curried Tuna Salad

Tuna Quinoa Cakes

Lean and Green Meal:

Pork Loin with Tomatoes and Olives

Day 7:

Fueling Hacks:

Baked Kale Chips

Grilled Buffalo Shrimp

Cranberry Sweet Potato Muffins

Buckwheat Crepes

Oatmeal Pancakes

Lean and Green Meal:

Cauliflower Ground Beef Hash

Week 3

Day 1:

Fueling Hacks:

Cranberry Sweet Potato Muffins

Baked Kale Chips

Grilled Buffalo Shrimp

Buckwheat Crepes

Oatmeal Pancakes

Lean and Green Meal:

Seared Scallops

Day 2:

Fueling Hacks:

Celery Salad

Yogurt Trail Mix Bars

Quinoa Pudding

Curried Tuna Salad

Tuna Quinoa Cakes

Lean and Green Meal:

Turkey Taco Soup

Day 3:

Fueling Hacks:

Taco Salad

Cranberry Sweet Potato Muffins

Quinoa Bars

Yogurt Trail Mix Bars

Oatmeal Pancakes

Lean and Green Meal:

Creamy Scallops

Day 4:

Fueling Hacks:

Buckwheat Crepes

Baked Kale Chips

Grilled Buffalo Shrimp

Celery Salad

Curried Tuna Salad

Tuna Quinoa Cakes

Lean and Green Meal:

Mojo Marinated Flank Steak

Day 5:

Fueling Hacks:

Quinoa Pudding

Yogurt Trail Mix Bars

Curried Tuna Salad

Tuna Quinoa Cakes

Lean and Green Meal:

Poached Mahi Mahi

Day 6:

Fueling Hacks:

Celery Salad

Baked Kale Chips

Grilled Buffalo Shrimp

Curried Tuna Salad

Cranberry Sweet Potato Muffins

Lean and Green Meal:

Pork Loin with Tomatoes and Olives

Day 7:

Fueling Hacks:

Cranberry Sweet Potato Muffins

Quinoa Bars

Tuna Quinoa Cakes

Buckwheat Crepes

Yogurt Trail Mix Bars

Lean and Green Meal:

Cauliflower Ground Beef Hash

Week 4

Day 1:

Fueling Hacks:

Quinoa Pudding

Cranberry Sweet Potato Muffins

Baked Kale Chips

Grilled Buffalo Shrimp

Oatmeal Pancakes

Lean and Green Meal:

Seared Scallops

Day 2:

Fueling Hacks:

Quinoa Pudding

Celery Salad

Taco Salad

Yogurt Trail Mix Bars

Tuna Quinoa Cakes

Lean and Green Meal:

Turkey Taco Soup

Day 3:

Fueling Hacks:

Curried Tuna Salad

Cranberry Sweet Potato Muffins

Quinoa Bars

Buckwheat Crepes

Celery Salad

Lean and Green Meal:

Creamy Scallops

Day 4:

Fueling Hacks:

Oatmeal Pancakes

Baked Kale Chips

Grilled Buffalo Shrimp

Curried Tuna Salad

Celery Salad

Lean and Green Meal:

Mojo Marinated Flank Steak

Day 5:

Fueling Hacks:

Tuna Quinoa Cakes

Taco Salad

Yogurt Trail Mix Bars

Curried Tuna Salad

Tuna Quinoa Cakes

Lean and Green Meal:

Poached Mahi Mahi

Day 6:

Fueling Hacks:

Yogurt Trail Mix Bars

Celery Salad

Taco Salad

Curried Tuna Salad

Tuna Quinoa Cakes

Lean and Green Meal:

Pork Loin with Tomatoes and Olives

Day 7:

Fueling Hacks:

Baked Kale Chips

Grilled Buffalo Shrimp

Cranberry Sweet Potato Muffins

Buckwheat Crepes

Oatmeal Pancakes

Lean and Green Meal:

Cauliflower Ground Beef Hash

4, 2 & 1 Meal Pan

Week 1

Day 1:

Fueling Hacks:

Quinoa Bars

Taco Cups

Caprese Spaghetti Squash Nests

Buckwheat Crepes

Lean and Green Meals:

Green Chicken Casserole

Salmon Chowder

Snack:

½ cup peaches

Day 2:

Fueling Hacks:

Tuna Quinoa Cakes

Taco Salad

Yogurt Trail Mix Bars

Curried Tuna Salad

Lean and Green Meals:

Sesame Chicken

Pork With Caramelized Mushrooms

Snack:

¾ cup low-fat plain yogurt

Day 3:

Fueling Hacks:

Fire Cracker Shrimp

Crispy Zucchini Chips

Quinoa Bars

Buckwheat Crepes

Lean and Green Meals:

Spinach Mushroom Chicken

Sirloin with Horseradish Sauce

Snack:

4 ounces apple

Day 4:

Fueling Hacks:

Yogurt Trail Mix Bars

Crispy Zucchini Chips

Taco Salad

Tuna Quinoa Cakes

Lean and Green Meals:

Chicken Piccata

Chipotle Pork Loin

Snack:

3 celery stalks

Day 5:

Fueling Hacks:

Cranberry Sweet Potato Muffins

Quinoa Pudding

Quinoa Bars

Buckwheat Crepes

Lean and Green Meals:

Chicken with Avocado Salsa

Cauliflower Ground Beef Hash

Snack:

½ cup fresh strawberries

Day 6:

Fueling Hacks:

Curried Tuna Salad

Taco Salad

Yogurt Trail Mix Bars

Crispy Zucchini Chips

Lean and Green Meals:

Broccoli Chicken Casserole

Pork Tenderloins with Mushrooms

Snack:

1 cup unsweetened cashew milk

Day 7:

Fueling Hacks:

Quinoa Bars

Crispy Zucchini Chips

Cranberry Sweet Potato Muffins

Buckwheat Crepes

Lean and Green Meals:

Chicken with Green Beans

Pork Loin with Tomatoes and Olives

Snack:

4 ounces orange

Week 2

Day 1:

Fueling Hacks:

Yogurt Trail Mix Bars

Crispy Zucchini Chips

Curried Tuna Salad

Tuna Quinoa Cakes

Lean and Green Meals:

Cheddar Turkey Burgers

Shrimp Pineapple

Snack:

½ cup peaches

Day 2:

Fueling Hacks:

Quinoa Pudding

Buckwheat Crepes

Crispy Zucchini Chips

Quinoa Bars

Lean and Green Meals:

Turkey Taco Soup

Grilled salmon with Avocado Salsa

Snack:

¾ cup low-fat plain yogurt

Day 3:

Fueling Hacks:

Crispy Zucchini Chips

Taco Salad

Yogurt Trail Mix Bars

Curried Tuna Salad

Lean and Green Meals:

Chicken Zucchini

Herb Roasted Tenderloin

Snack:

4 ounces apple

Day 4:

Fueling Hacks:

Buckwheat Crepes

Quinoa Pudding

Cranberry Sweet Potato Muffins

Crispy Zucchini Chips

Lean and Green Meals:

Turkey Shepherds Pie

Lamb Cabbage Rolls

Snack:

3 celery stalks

Day 5:

Fueling Hacks:

Yogurt Trail Mix Bars

Taco Salad

Curried Tuna Salad

Tuna Quinoa Cakes

Lean and Green Meals:

Turkey Broccoli

Shrimp Salad

Snack:

½ cup fresh strawberries

Day 6:

Fueling Hacks:

Cranberry Sweet Potato Muffins

Crispy Zucchini Chips

Quinoa Bars

Buckwheat Crepes

Lean and Green Meals:

Baked Chicken Stuffed

Pan Seared Beef and Mushrooms

Snack:

1 cup unsweetened cashew milk

Day 7:

Fueling Hacks:

Curried Tuna Salad

Taco Salad

Crispy Zucchini Chips

Tuna Quinoa Cakes

Lean and Green Meals:

Stuffed Chicken Breast

Halibut With Zucchini Noodles

Snack:

4 ounces orange

Week 3

Day 1:

Fueling Hacks:

Quinoa Bars

Taco Cups

Caprese Spaghetti Squash Nests

Buckwheat Crepes

Lean and Green Meals:

Green Chicken Casserole

Salmon Chowder

Snack:

½ cup peaches

Day 2:

Fueling Hacks:

Tuna Quinoa Cakes

Taco Salad

Yogurt Trail Mix Bars

Curried Tuna Salad

Lean and Green Meals:

Sesame Chicken

Pork With Caramelized Mushrooms

Snack:

¾ cup low-fat plain yogurt

Day 3:

Fueling Hacks:

Fire Cracker Shrimp

Crispy Zucchini Chips

Quinoa Bars

Buckwheat Crepes

Lean and Green Meals:

Spinach Mushroom Chicken

Sirloin with Horseradish Sauce

Snack:

4 ounces apple

Day 4:

Fueling Hacks:

Yogurt Trail Mix Bars

Crispy Zucchini Chips

Taco Salad

Tuna Quinoa Cakes

Lean and Green Meals:

Chicken Piccata

Chipotle Pork Loin

Snack:

3 celery stalks

Day 5:

Fueling Hacks:

Cranberry Sweet Potato Muffins

Quinoa Pudding

Quinoa Bars

Buckwheat Crepes

Lean and Green Meals:

Chicken with Avocado Salsa

Cauliflower Ground Beef Hash

Snack:

½ cup fresh strawberries

Day 6:

Fueling Hacks:

Curried Tuna Salad

Taco Salad

Yogurt Trail Mix Bars

Crispy Zucchini Chips

Lean and Green Meals:

Broccoli Chicken Casserole

Pork Tenderloins with Mushrooms

Snack:

1 cup unsweetened cashew milk

Day 7:

Fueling Hacks:

Quinoa Bars

Crispy Zucchini Chips

Cranberry Sweet Potato Muffins

Buckwheat Crepes

Lean and Green Meals:

Chicken with Green Beans

Pork Loin with Tomatoes and Olives

Snack:

4 ounces orange

Week 4

Day 1:

Fueling Hacks:

Yogurt Trail Mix Bars

Crispy Zucchini Chips

Curried Tuna Salad

Tuna Quinoa Cakes

Lean and Green Meals:

Cheddar Turkey Burgers

Shrimp Pineapple

Snack:

½ cup peaches

Day 2:

Fueling Hacks:

Quinoa Pudding

Buckwheat Crepes

Crispy Zucchini Chips

Quinoa Bars

Lean and Green Meals:

Turkey Taco Soup

Grilled salmon with Avocado Salsa

Snack:

¾ cup low-fat plain yogurt

Day 3:

Fueling Hacks:

Crispy Zucchini Chips

Taco Salad

Yogurt Trail Mix Bars

Curried Tuna Salad

Lean and Green Meals:

Chicken Zucchini

Herb Roasted Tenderloin

Snack:

4 ounces apple

Day 4:

Fueling Hacks:

Buckwheat Crepes

Quinoa Pudding

Cranberry Sweet Potato Muffins

Crispy Zucchini Chips

Lean and Green Meals:

Turkey Shepherds Pie

Lamb Cabbage Rolls

Snack:

3 celery stalks

Day 5:

Fueling Hacks:

Yogurt Trail Mix Bars

Taco Salad

Curried Tuna Salad

Tuna Quinoa Cakes

Lean and Green Meals:

Turkey Broccoli

Shrimp Salad

Snack:

½ cup fresh strawberries

Day 6:

Fueling Hacks:

Cranberry Sweet Potato Muffins

Crispy Zucchini Chips

Quinoa Bars

Buckwheat Crepes

Lean and Green Meals:

Baked Chicken Stuffed

Pan Seared Beef and Mushrooms

Snack:

1 cup unsweetened cashew milk

Day 7:

Fueling Hacks:

Curried Tuna Salad

Taco Salad

Crispy Zucchini Chips

Tuna Quinoa Cakes

Lean and Green Meals:

Stuffed Chicken Breast

Halibut With Zucchini Noodles

Snack:

4 ounces orange

Conclusion

Are you ready to shed some pounds using the lean and green diet? Well, the whole approach mainly functions around the concept of calorie restriction. When you reduce your caloric intake, the body starts breaking down the existing reserves of glycogen and fats in the body to meet its need. This gradually helps in losing weight. According to the lean and green diet, the caloric intake should be around 1000 calories per day in order to initiate fat burning in the body. Since all diet plans suggesting such a drastic calorie cutdown omits a lot of food from the menu. You need to give up on a lot of things to keep your caloric intake this low. And this struggle of cutting down calories on a daily basis makes a dieter quit sooner than he planned to.

The lean and green diet, on the other hand, provides a perfect solution. It is easy and simple to follow because it offers the use of special powdered food known as fueling, which is made specially to keep the calories low and provide all the essential nutrients that are required to carry out the normal metabolic activities in the body. In simple words, it offers weight loss with good health, and you can manage to live on this diet without the fear of suffering from malnutrition or any nutritional deficiency. Each fueling is created to have only 100 to 110 calories, which is low enough to keep the daily caloric intake to 1000 calories.

Besides cutting down the caloric intake through the use of special fueling, the lean and green diet also aids weight loss through its "Lean and Green" meals. The diet is not all about Fuelings; rather, it gives you different options to enjoy actual food and its different flavors as well. As long as you are following the plan and eating lean and green food, you can expect to lose weight. It's about time that you put these recipes and the meal plan to practical use! Opt for this diet plan and see its claimed benefits yourself. You will be surprised by the results!

CPSIA information can be obtained
at www.ICGtesting.com
Printed in the USA
BVHW061011130421
604814BV00008B/1413